Epilepsy and Pregnancy

Epilepsy and Pregnancy

Edited by

TORBJÖRN TOMSON

Department of Clinical Neuroscience, Karolinska Hospital, Stockholm, Sweden

LENNART GRAM

Department of Neurology, State University Hospital, Copenhagen, Denmark

MATTI SILLANPÄÄ

Department of Child Neurology, University of Turku Hospital, Finland

SVEIN I. JOHANNESSEN

The National Center for Epilepsy, Sandvika, Norway

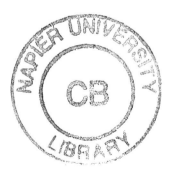

WRIGHTSON BIOMEDICAL PUBLISHING LTD
Petersfield, UK and Bristol, PA, USA

Editorial Office:

Wrightson Biomedical Publishing Ltd
Ash Barn House, Winchester Road, Stroud,
Petersfield, Hampshire GU32 3PN, UK
Telephone: 01730 265647
Fax: 01730 260368

British Library Cataloguing in Publication Data
Epilepsy and pregnancy
   1. Epilepsy 2. Epilepsy – Genetic aspects 3. Epilepsy in
pregnancy
   I. Tomson, Torbjorn
   616.8'53

Library of Congress Cataloging in Publication Data
Epilepsy and pregnancy / edited by Torbjörn Tomson ... et al ...
   p. cm.
  Includes bibliographical references and index.
  ISBN 1-871816-36-X (hard cover)
  1. Epilepsy in pregnancy. I. Tomson, Torbjörn, 1950–
  [DNLM: 1. Epilepsy—in pregnancy. 2. Epilepsy—drug therapy.
  3. Anticonvulsants—therapeutic use. 4. Pregnancy Complications.
  WL 385 E604 1997]
  RG580.E64E63 1997
  618.3—dc21
  DNLM/DLC
  for Library of Congress   97–9933
                                     CIP

ISBN 1 871816 36 X

Composition by Scribe Design, Gillingham, Kent
Printed in Great Britain by Biddles Ltd, Guildford.

Contents

Contributors

Bengt R. Danielsson, *Astra Safety Assessment, S-151 85 Södertälje, and Department of Pharmaceutical Biosciences, Division of Toxicology, Uppsala University, S-751 24 Uppsala, Sweden*

Lennart Dencker, *Department of Pharmaceutical Biosciences, Division of Toxicology, Uppsala University, S-751 24 Uppsala, Sweden*

Wiggo Fischer-Rasmussen, *Department of Obstetrics and Gynaecology, Hvidovre Hospital, University of Copenhagen, DK-2650 Hvidovre, Denmark*

Mogens Laue Friis, *Department of Neurology, Odense University Hospital, DK-5000 Odense C, Denmark*

Eija Gaily, *Department of Child Neurology, University of Helsinki, Children's Castle Hospital, Lastenlinnantie 2, FIN-00250 Helsinki, Finland*

R. Mark Gardiner, *Department of Paediatrics, University College London Medical School, The Rayne Institute, 5 University Street, London WC1E 6JJ, UK*

Lennart Gram, *Department of Neurology, State University Hospital, DK-2100 Copenhagen, Denmark*

Vilho Hiilesmaa, *Department of Obstetrics and Gynaecology, Helsinki University, FIN-00290 Helsinki, Finland*

Svein I. Johannessen, *The National Center for Epilepsy, N-1301 Sandvika, Norway*

Anna-Elina Lehesjoki, *Department of Medical Genetics, University of Helsinki, FIN-00014 Helsinki, Finland*

Dick Lindhout, *MGC-Department of Clinical Genetics, Erasmus University, PO Box 1738, 3000 DR Rotterdam, The Netherlands*

Heinz Nau, *Department of Food Toxicology, Centre of Food Sciences, Veterinary Medical University, Bischofsholer Damm 15, D-30173 Hannover, Germany*

Leena Peltonen, *National Public Health Institute and Institute of Biomedicine, Department of Human Molecular Genetics, University of Helsinki, FIN-00300 Helsinki, Finland*

Anders Rane, *Department of Clinical Pharmacology, University Hospital, S-751 85 Uppsala, Sweden*

Anne Sabers, *Department of Neurology, State University Hospital, DK-2100 Copenhagen, Denmark*

E. Bettina Samrén, *MGC-Department of Clinical Genetics, Erasmus University, PO Box 1738, 3000 DR Rotterdam, The Netherlands*

Matti Sillanpää, *Department of Paediatric Neurology, University of Turku Hospital TYKS, FIN-20520 Turku, Finland*

Per Sjöberg, *Division of Pharmacology and Toxicology, Medical Products Agency, S-521 24 Uppsala, Sweden*

Torbjörn Tomson, *Department of Clinical Neuroscience, Division of Neurology, Karolinska Hospital, S-171 76 Stockholm, Sweden*

Ellen Vinge, *Department of Clinical Pharmacology, Lund University Hospital, S-221 85 Lund, Sweden*

Foreword

During the past three to four decades, reproductive issues in epilepsy have attracted increasingly more attention. It started with publications in the early 1960s, with reports on pregnancy outcome in women taking antiepileptic drugs like phenytoin, phenobarbitone, or primidone, or the anticonvulsive medication diazepam. Reports on single cases and case series describing co-occurrence or associations between prenatal antiepileptic drug exposures and major malformations, minor anomalies, pre- and postnatal growth retardation, or mental developmental deficiencies raised concern about the safety of antiepileptic medication to the human fetus. Initially, most of these studies were based on retrospective data, or derived from patient populations that were selected for special types of epilepsy care or fetal outcome, and they did not control for maternal seizure and epilepsy characteristics, or genetic factors in general. Subsequently, several groups started prospective studies, based on less select patient populations, and made comparisons between various medications or with control pregnancies.

The current volume on *Epilepsy and Pregnancy* not only reflects the results of research conducted over the past 15 years, and the major contributions made by Nordic groups, but also confronts us with many new and important challenges for the coming decade.

The first challenge is the rapid and reliable evaluation of the teratogenic potential of the 10 or so new antiepileptic drugs which have been developed over the past 10 years and which are now being released for prescription in many countries. Some of these drugs showed teratogenic effects in animal experiments. Others did not, which, in view of extensive interspecies susceptibility, does not exclude teratogenicity in human pregnancies. This book explores the factors that play a role in balancing the pros and cons of use of new versus old compounds in the pharmacological treatment of women of reproductive age with epilepsy, and stresses the demand for collaborative research and postmarketing surveillance programmes of pregnancies with antiepileptic drug use on a population basis.

A second challenge is the molecular genetic analysis of the aetiologies and pathogenetic mechanisms of epilepsy. This issue summarizes the recent breakthroughs in localization and identification of genes for epilepsy syndromes with monogenic inheritance, and provides reviews of methods that have been successfully applied in several other common diseases with complex aetiology. This kind of research needs, again, multidisciplinary and international collaboration. The outcome of these studies will improve our ability to counsel epilepsy patients who wish to have children, and help in the development of new treatment and prevention strategies. Finally, they will also allow us to sort out the contributions made by *nature* and *nurture* in the teratological issues.

The third challenge is to translate the results of this research into improved health care and better counselling of patients and relatives. For many decades there has been a taboo about reproduction and reproductive issues in epilepsy. The present volume makes it clear that attitudes have changed, and that challenges for the near future have been identified with success. This book concludes with well-balanced recommendations with respect to counselling and treatment of women of reproductive age, during pregnancy, and around delivery. Detailed considerations are given to primary prevention by adjustment of medication and periconceptional folic acid supplementation, and about secondary prevention by various means of prenatal diagnosis. Most patients with epilepsy can have healthy children, provided that appropriate counselling and health care is given, and that the teratogenic side-effects of new drugs are identified and estimated as early as possible.

DICK LINDHOUT
Chairman,
ILAE Commission on Genetics, Pregnancy, and the Child

Preface

To form a family and have children is one of the most important aspects of a normal life. Yet, not so long ago, people with epilepsy were denied this fundamental right in many parts of the world including the Scandinavian countries, prevented by prejudiced legislation. Fortunately, the situation has changed radically over the past few decades, and more and more women with epilepsy become pregnant and have children. It has been estimated that 0.3–0.4% of all children today are born to mothers with epilepsy. The pregnancy of a woman with epilepsy may, however, be more complicated than that of a healthy woman. Antiepileptic drug treatment increases the risk of birth defects, and the rate of obstetric complications is higher. In addition, pregnancy may affect seizure control and alter the pharmacokinetics of antiepileptic drugs. Even breast-feeding may be complicated by the mother's use of antiepileptic drugs. The recent introduction of several new antiepileptic drugs has added to the complexity of this issue.

The risk to the child of inheriting the mother's or the father's epilepsy is another important topic. The genetic aspects of epilepsy are therefore an important issue in any discussion of epilepsy and pregnancy.

Clearly, epilepsy in pregnancy represents a challenge both to basic science and clinical research, and a close collaboration between toxicologists, teratologists, pharmacologists, geneticists, and neuroscientists is essential in order to extend our knowledge. Likewise, a multidisciplinary effort engaging neurologists, neonatologists, paediatricians, obstetricians, and clinical pharmacologists is necessary to achieve optimal management of the pregnant woman with epilepsy.

The purpose of this volume is to present an up-to-date overview of all the clinically relevant aspects of the management and care of the woman with epilepsy. The book is intended for neurologists, paediatricians, paediatric neurologists, obstetricians, general practitioners, and other professionals who are engaged in the treatment of women with epilepsy, or involved in the care of their offspring. A further objective is to stimulate collaborative research efforts in order to advance our knowledge. The volume presents primarily the view of Scandinavian experts, but includes contributions from German, Dutch and British researchers. The reader is given an introductory overview of developmental toxicology and teratology, and the reliability of methods of preclinical screening methods for teratogenic effects is debated. The pharmacokinetics of antiepileptic drugs in the pregnant woman, the fetus and the neonate are reviewed, along with a survey of the issues concerning breast-feeding while taking antiepileptic drugs. Complications during pregnancy are reviewed and the potential methods of reducing them discussed. Further, methods for prenatal diagnosis of malformations are presented.

The application of new methods in genetic studies is likely to have implications beyond genetic counselling, and may increase our understanding of the molecular mechanisms underlying epilepsy. Several chapters are therefore devoted to genetics, introducing the methodology of molecular genetics and presenting the most recent advances in the genetics of epilepsy.

The topics were suggested by the Editors, but the content of each contribution is entirely the author's. However, in an attempt to form a synthesis of the facts and opinions presented in the various chapters, the Editors present their recommendations for counselling, management and care of pregnant women with epilepsy at the end of this volume.

The Editors would like to express their gratitude to all the authors for their contributions, to Ciba in Denmark, Finland, Norway and Sweden for educational grants, and to Lars-Ove Zetterlöf, Rauli Laaksonen, Arvid Lian and Benedikte Østergaard, for their invaluable assistance in the preparation of this publication.

THE EDITORS

1

Fetal Development and Sensitivity Periods in Man

LENNART DENCKER

Department of Pharmaceutical Biosciences, Uppsala University, Uppsala, Sweden

INTRODUCTION

The purpose of this chapter is to give a broad review of important developmental events related to the most commonly occurring or retrospectively important malformations induced by exogenous insults to the human embryo/fetus. Due to the abundance of excellent illustrated textbooks on human embryology, no illustrations will be presented here. Several data have been taken from Larsen (1993).

From a clinical and toxicological point of view, the risks of drug-induced malformations have received considerable attention. In general, side-effects of drugs may arise from exaggerated pharmacology, secondary pharmacology (i.e. undesired pharmacological effects), hypersensitivity and allergic reactions, and direct toxicity. The latter is quite often caused by the production of toxic intermediates by biotransformation and, in general terms, and with all other factors kept constant, there is a relation between dose and toxicity. With the development of more potent drugs the doses given to patients (and thus tissue concentrations) tend to decrease, and consequently so does the number of molecules available for the undesired biotransformation or other expressions of nonspecific toxicity.

Although in this way side-effects of drugs in general may decrease, the risk of fetal toxicity may not necessarily do so. It is true that mechanisms of fetal toxicity and the induction of malformations are not well known, but obviously undesired pharmacological effects are often involved, and these will be difficult to avoid unless drugs can be designed which do not pass into the embryonic/fetal circulation (so far, wishful thinking only).

Some important determinants or principles in developmental toxicology, many of which will be dealt with in this volume, are the significance of (1) genotype; (2) developmental stage when an insult takes place;

1

(3) mechanisms of action; (4) pharmacokinetics of the drug in the mother and conceptus; (5) the manifestations of embryo/fetotoxicity such as death, malformations, growth inhibition and functional disturbances; and (6) dose–effect and dose–response relationships. This chapter will deal mainly with the developmental events and their significance for stage-specific sensitivity of the embryo/fetus. For the interested reader, an excellent textbook chapter on developmental toxicology is available (Rogers and Kavlock, 1996).

HOW CAN WE OBTAIN INFORMATION ON SENSITIVITY PERIODS?

It is possible to find some clues as to when an organ is most sensitive to exogenous agents that cause or are suspected of causing teratogenic effects, simply by consulting a textbook on embryology. For example, a cleft palate cannot be induced by drugs administered beyond approximately day 60 after conception, when the palate is closed. By studying the nature of a malformation, it is also to some extent possible to define the period when the insult must have been made.

Today there is an increasing amount of data from experimental animals (mostly the mouse) on tissue- and stage-specific gene expression during development. Since there are relatively good comparisons on developmental stages between human and animal embryos, it will increasingly be possible in future to anticipate when genes of regulatory importance may be expressed also in the human embryo. Thus, if we deal with drugs (such as retinoids), known to affect directly or indirectly the expression of specific genes regulating pattern formation or related events in the embryo, then we may by inference calculate corresponding sensitivity periods in human embryos. In addition, drugs not known to affect genes directly may, by nonspecifically disturbing cell function, shift a well orchestrated gene expression pattern and thus cause malformations.

However promising for the future, so far we have very little specific information on drug interaction with genes regulating development, or, for that matter, interaction with other molecules of developmental interest. Some well investigated drugs will, however, be dealt with in a later section of this chapter.

IMPORTANT DEVELOPMENTAL EVENTS

Preimplantation

After fertilization, the conceptus develops by cleavage and formation of a blastocyst, which is implanted into the uterine endometrium at around day 6.5. During this period the conceptus of experimental animals has traditionally, with a few exceptions, been considered refractory to exogenous insults in terms of induction of classical malformations. A reasonable explanation for this may be that if a massive insult occurs during this developmental stage it will kill the conceptus, while if only a few cells are damaged they may be replaced, since the cells still maintain a high degree of pluripotency. In mice, it has been possible to induce tail and hind leg duplications by administering retinoic acid in the late preimplantation period (days 4.5–5.5; gastrulation begins on day 6.5 in the mouse). Spina bifida was typically induced at day 6, and eye defects at day 7 (Rutledge et al., 1994). Although not of immediate clinical relevance, these early retinoic-acid-induced caudal duplications again show that very early differentiation events may be influenced. This whole problem is for several reasons difficult to study in women, one reason being that a high percentage of embryos are in any case lost in the first period of pregnancy due to genetic/chromosomal anomalies. Another reason is the difficulty of reconstructing exactly, day by day, when a drug may have been administered relative to the embryonic stage.

Genomic imprinting is an epigenetic phenomenon by which the two parental alleles of a gene are differentially expressed depending on whether they are of maternal origin (mainly contributing to embryonic development), or paternal origin (contributing to the placenta). Although the function of genomic imprinting is not clear, it has been proposed that it evolved in mammals to regulate intrauterine growth (Leighton et al., 1996). Toxicity to imprinting could conceivably play a role during the first week of gestation, as well as in, for example, paternally mediated developmental toxicity (Olshan and Mattison, 1995).

Second to third weeks

During this period, gastrulation (formation of the three germ layers) and beginning of placental formation takes place. At this stage the ectoderm receives important inductive signals from the underlying axial mesoderm to form the neural plate. It has been shown in mice that, when administered during gastrulation, ethanol and retinoic acid cause a major insult to the anterior neural plate, which results in characteristic ocular, brain and facial malformations, for ethanol comparable to those seen in fetal alcohol syndrome in human babies (Sulik et al., 1988). A syndrome known as caudal dysplasia (caudal regression) is considered to be induced during the third week and to be due to defects in growth and migration of mesoderm.

Components of the caudal dysplasia syndrome are strongly overrepresented among children born to diabetic mothers (however, a very rare syndrome), and corresponding malformations can also be induced in early gestation in diabetic rats (Eriksson et al., 1989), consistent with an influence during the gastrulation period.

Table 1. Some developmental events during the organogenetic period of human development (days after conception).

Day	Event
20	First somites formed; neuromers in brain vesicles
22	Neural folds begin to fuse; heart begins to pump; first two pharyngeal arches
24	Cranial neuropore closes; optic vesicles and optic pits develop
26	Caudal neuropore closes; pharyngeal arches 3 and 4 form; upper limb buds appear
28	Lower limb buds appear; ureteric buds appear; lens placodes appear
32	Spinal nerves begin to sprout; metanephros begins to appear; intestinal loops form; lens invaginates in optic cup; cerebral hemispheres begin to form
33	Genital tubercles appear; atrioventricular valves form; medial and lateral nasal processes visible; sensory and parasympathetic nerve ganglia and olfactory neurons visible
37	Muscular ventricular septum forms; kidney calyces form and kidneys start to ascend; genital ridges appear; foot plates form; pigment in retina pigment epithelium
41	Septum intermedium in heart completed; finger rays are distinct; cerebellum begins to form; melanocytes in dermis
44	Skeletal ossification begins; Sertoli cells differentiate; toe rays appear; eyelids form; thalami and diencephalon expand; nipples and hair follicles appear
50	Upper limbs bend at elbows; vasa deferens begin to form; primary intestinal loop completed
56–58	Palatal closure

The organogenetic period

This is the period (approximately days 21–56; Table 1) when the fetus is considered most sensitive to the induction by exogenous agents of classical malformations in single organs and/or syndromes of malformations. Differentiating cells in various organ *anlagen* now start to develop susceptibility, for example, to drugs affecting specific receptors. This is also a period of extensive cell migration, morphogenetic movements, cell–cell and cell–matrix interactions, and so on. Crucial developmental events are presented in Table 1. Known human teratogens which are active mostly in this period are cytostatics, isotretinoin, thalidomide, diethylstilboestrol, valproic acid (spina bifida), warfarin, as regards its tendency to induce embryopathy (as opposed to bleedings later in gestation), and ethanol, with respect to facial dysmorphogenesis, for example.

The fetal period

Exposure in this period (after the eighth week) is not considered to result in major morphological malformations. However, it should be made clear that development is a continuum, in the fetal as well as in the embryonic period. Moreover, any particular drug may affect processes in the embryonic as well as in the fetal period. Receptors and other molecular drug targets for functions to come are continuously developing, making the fetus possibly even more sensitive than the embryo to some pharmacological agents/effects. Thus, the use of angiotensin converting enzyme (ACE) inhibitors in the second and third trimesters may be associated with a high degree of fetal and newborn morbidity, and even mortality, due to disturbance of regulatory mechanisms of the fetal blood pressure leading to kidney and skull malformations, in addition to oligo/anuria and oligohydramniosis. Some authors recommend that the use of drugs in this group should be avoided at all trimesters of pregnancy (Shotan *et al.*, 1994). In addition, the new generation of drugs affecting the angiotensin system, the angiotensin II receptor antagonists (e.g. Losartan), tend to induce fetotoxicity and fetal kidney damage in experimental animals, indicating in principle a similar mechanism of action to that of the ACE inhibitors.

Warfarin is considered to cause facial dysmorphogenesis when administered in the first trimester, the critical period being weeks 6–9 of gestation (reviewed by Howe and Webster, 1992). Haemorrhages of the central nervous system, on the other hand, occur after second and third trimester exposure. Animal experiments have elegantly demonstrated that the mechanisms behind the two types of malformation are different. It is proposed that the facial features of the human warfarin embryopathy are caused by reduced growth of the embryonic nasal septum, which occurs not because of bleeding (warfarin-sensitive clotting factors have not yet developed), but because the warfarin-induced extrahepatic vitamin K deficiency prevents the normal formation of the vitamin K-dependent gamma-carboxyglutamic acid containing (gla) protein matrix in the embryonic cartilage (Howe and Webster, 1992).

SOME HUMAN TERATOGENS OF SPECIAL INTEREST

Isotretinoin

Isotretinoin is a retinoid, 13-*cis*-retinoic acid, which has been used as an oral anti-acne drug for more than 10 years. It is a human teratogen which most probably functions by isomerizing in the body to all-trans retinoic acid, which has been studied extensively as an experimental teratogen (Nau *et al.*, 1994; Means and Gudas, 1995, and references therein). While, in experimental animals, malformations can be induced in several organs, in human embryos the central nervous system, notably hindbrain derivatives (especially brainstem, cerebellum and cranial nerves) and neural crest cell derivatives (face, external ears, thymus and heart/great vessels causing aortico-pulmonary septation defects) is disturbed. This syndrome of malformations is consistent with an effect in the period of hindbrain segmentation, which starts around day 20 in the human embryo. Combined with the collective information from a vast literature from cell culture systems to whole animal experiments, the human malformations indicate that the important Hox gene family, being expressed in a time- and space-restricted manner in the hindbrain at these stages of development, is regulated by retinoic acid via its nuclear receptors (Means and Gudas, 1995). It also indicates that these genes, involved in the process of laying down the fundamental segmentation pattern of the hindbrain, are the most easily disturbed of all genes important during the organogenetic period (in terms of dose–effect relationships) by overdosing this naturally occurring receptor ligand in the form of a pharmaceutical product. Isotretinoin exposure during the first trimester poses a risk of around 25% for major malformations and, in addition, a high risk of sponta- neous abortion, premature delivery and developmental disabilities (Nau *et al.*, 1994, and references therein).

Thalidomide

Thalidomide was shown to affect limb development in a time-restricted manner, days 20–36 after conception being the approximate sensitivity period, the upper limb being affected earlier than the lower limb. Already the early limb bud has a regional diversification, and the expression pattern of some genes co-localize with classically defined 'signal centres', long since known to direct pattern formation of the limb. Such centres are the zone of polarizing activity (ZPA), the apical ectodermal ridge (AER), and the progressive zone (see Johnson *et al.*, 1994, for review). The progressive zone comprises the dividing cells of the mesenchyme underneath the AER, which leave in a proximal direction to contribute to more proximal skeletal elements. Since the cells giving rise to presumptive proximal limb structure leave first, it is to be expected that thalidomide, which tended to affect proxi- mal structures more than distal ones (except thumb), affects the very earli- est stages of limb development.

Thalidomide also induced malformations in other structures such as the ear and cranial nerves, indicative of damage in the fourth week (Miller and Strömland, 1991). This time-limited effect again strongly indicates that thalidomide affects specific molecules involved in early pattern formation as described for isotretinoin.

Ethanol

There is intriguing evidence from studies in mice (see above) as well as non- human primates that the appearance of the frontonasal complex in fetal alcohol syndrome (FAS) may be caused by an influence very early in development (gastrulation and early organogenetic period, the third and fourth weeks), and that it in fact represents a mild form of holoprosencephaly (Sulik *et al.*, 1988; Siebert *et al.*, 1991). Combined human and animal experimental data also indicate that some of the central nervous system (CNS) and eye malformations (e.g. atrophy of the optic nerve; Strömland, personal communication, 1995) may be induced as early as weeks 3–5 after conception. The most likely nonspecific mechanisms of action of ethanol and its major toxic metabolite, acetaldehyde, however, suggest that the embryo/fetus can be sensitive throughout the whole period of intrauterine development, including the brain growth spurt in the last trimester.

Antiepileptic drugs

These drugs are the main theme of this volume, and will not be covered in this chapter. However, they have some characteristics in common with ethanol, for example, that they are often consumed throughout pregnancy and may thus, in principle, affect most developmental processes provided that they have the biochemical prerequisite for doing so. The partly differential patterns of malformations induced by the individual antiepileptics, however, indicate substance-related effects, e.g. spina bifida for valproic acid (see Chapter 4), and substance-specific changes in the facial appearance. An interesting mechanism of action put forward recently is the effect of several antiepileptics on the cardiovascular system, favouring common mechanisms not only for a group of antiepileptics but for several other teratogenic factors (see Chapter 3). The resulting malformations, for example of apical structures such as fingers, show that malformations may occur also after the strict organogenetic period.

Diethylstilboestrol (DES)

Exposure of pregnant women to the nonsteroidal oestrogen DES has caused several types of reproductive aberrations and dysfunctions in both female and male offspring. Vaginal epithelial changes (adenosis), sometimes transformed into adenocarcinomas after puberty, were the most frequent if the embryo was exposed before the eighth week of gestation (Herbst, 1992).

Miscellaneous

Most modern drug compendia (such as the *Farmaceutical Specialities in Sweden* (FASS)) list drugs that are known to cause or are suspected of causing harmful effects to the fetus if administered to pregnant women. There is no reason to list them all in this chapter, only to give some general principles. As discussed above, the sensitivity period for any given drug may sometimes be reasonably well calculated from the type of insult observed, or the type of pharmacological effect the drug exerts. What should be remembered, however, is that only directly apparent morphological and physiological insults are recognized, while less is known about functional teratology, in experimental animals but especially in humans (for review, see several chapters in Kimmel and Buelke-Sam, 1994). The example given above for the DES disaster is one where a cancer appeared at a restricted age in the offspring (after puberty when this form of cancer is very rare in a normal population), which provided the impetus for functional studies on the reproductive tract of female as well as male offspring. An organ system such as the nervous system, which is in most respects difficult to test functionally, and has an extended period of development throughout pregnancy together with a considerable complexity, makes a determination of its sensitivity periods difficult.

CONCLUSIONS

This chapter has given some general views on sensitivity periods of the developing human embryo/fetus, exemplified by well-known teratogens. Focus has been placed on the first trimester, from which the majority of disasters of drug-related teratogenesis emanate, while the fetal period has been more superficially covered. This to some extent mirrors the greater clinical significance of early-induced damage to the offspring, but also the relative sparsity of information on more permanent changes induced by disturbances in the fetal period. In this period of development, pharmacological influence in fetal physiology may have been considered more or less reversible. This may, however, not necessarily be true. Future research may shed light on further interesting aspects of this problem.

REFERENCES

Eriksson, R.S.M., Thunberg, L. and Eriksson, U.J. (1989). Effects of interrupted insulin treatment on the fetal outcome of pregnant diabetic rats. *Diabetes* **38**, 764–722.

Herbst, A.L. (1992). *Long-Term Effects of Exposure to Diethylstilboestrol. NIH Workshop*. National Institute of Health, Falls Church, VA.

Howe, A.M. and Webster, W.S. (1992). The warfarin embryopathy: a rat model showing maxillonasal hypoplasia and other skeletal disturbances. *Teratology* **46**, 379–390.

Johnson, R.L., Riddle, R.D. and Tabin, C.J. (1994). Mechanisms of limb development. *Curr Biol* **4**, 535–542.

Kimmel, C.A. and Buelke-Sam, J. (Eds) (1994). *Developmental Toxicology 2nd edn.* Raven Press, New York.

Larsen, W.J. (1993). *Human Embryology*. Churchill Livingstone, Edinburgh.

Leighton, P.A., Saam, J.R., Ingram, R.S. and Tilghman, S.M. (1996). Genomic imprinting in mice: its function and mechanism. *Biol Reprod* **54**, 273–278.

Means, A.L. and Gudas, L.J. (1995). The roles of retinoids in vertebrate development. *Annu Rev Biochem* **64**, 201–233.

Miller, M.T. and Strömland, K. (1991). Ocular motility in thalidomide embryopathy. *J Pediatr Ophthalmol Strabismus* **28**, 47–54.

Nau, H., Chahoud, I., Dencker, L., Lammer, E.J. and Scott, W.J. (1994). Teratogenicity of vitamin A and retinoids. In: Blomhoff, R. (Ed.), *Vitamin A in Health and Disease*. Marcel Dekker, New York, pp. 615–663.

Olshan, A. and Mattison, D. (Eds) (1995). *Male-Mediated Developmental Toxicity*. Plenum Press, New York.

Rogers, J.M. and Kavlock, R.J. (1996). Developmental toxicology. In: Klassen, C.D. (Ed.), *Casarett & Doull's Toxicology: The Basic Science of Poisons*. McGraw-Hill, New York, pp. 301–331.

Rutledge, J.C., Shourbaji, A.G., Hughes, L.A. *et al.* (1994). Limb and lower-body duplications induced by retinoic acid in mice. *Proc Natl Acad Sci* **91**, 5436–5440.

Shotan, A., Widerhorn, J., Hurst, A. and Elkayam, U. (1994). Risks of anginotensin converting enzyme inhibition during pregnancy: experimental and clinical evidence, potential mechanisms, and recommendations for use. *Am J Med* **96**, 451–456.

Siebert, J.R., Astley, S.J. and Clarren, S.K. (1991). Holoprosencephaly in a fetal macaque (*Macaca nemestrina*) following weekly exposure to ethanol. *Teratology* **44**, 29–36.

Sulik, K.K., Cook, C.S. and Webster, W.S. (1988). Teratogens and craniofacial malformations: relationships to cell death. *Development* **103** (suppl), 213–231.

Epilepsy and Pregnancy
Edited by T. Tomson, L. Gram, M. Sillanpää and S.I. Johannessen
© 1997 Wrightson Biomedical Publishing Ltd

2

Preclinical Screening Methods and their Predictive Value

PER SJÖBERG

Division of Pharmacology and Toxicology, Medical Products Agency, Uppsala, Sweden

PRECLINICAL SCREENING METHODS

The evaluation of the potential of a new medicinal product to induce human developmental toxicity involves studies in pregnant animals. It is generally agreed that such studies should be conducted prior to any deliberate exposure of women of childbearing potential, although the US Food and Drug Administration may in certain circumstances allow the inclusion of these women in early and carefully controlled clinical trials. Recently developed *in vitro* methods, such as those utilizing mammalian organ or whole embryo culture techniques (Schmid, 1987), cannot replace *in vivo* animal testing, but could be used for screening purposes or for mechanistic studies.

As a result of the thalidomide catastrophe in the early 1960s, testing strategies in laboratory animals were developed to identify potential adverse effects during the embryonal, organogenesis and fetal periods (USFDA, 1966). In essence, these strategies are still advocated by drug regulatory authorities around the world. However, today there is also a focus on effects induced during the embryo-fetal period which become manifest postnatally. Recently, an expert working group under the auspices of the International Conference on Harmonization have refined the testing strategies and there is today a harmonized international guideline on the requirement for studies on toxicity to reproduction for pharmaceuticals in Japan, Europe and the United States (ICH, 1993).

Embryo-fetal toxicity, including teratogenicity, is normally assessed in two species such as the rat and the rabbit. The rat is also used to investigate effects which can only be detected postnatally such as physical development, sensory functions and reflexes and behaviour. Although the guideline states that 'if it can be shown that the species selected is a relevant model for the human, a single species can suffice', drug developers around the world normally take the safe approach and always perform studies in two species. When equivocal results are obtained, companies may use a third species such as the mouse or a non-human primate. These may also be the species of choice when the rat and/or the rabbit are found to be unsuitable.

Study design in rats and rabbits

Although several designs can be used to study the full spectrum of developmental toxic effects in the rat, the one which utilizes treatment from implantation (day 6 of gestation) to weaning could be regarded as the most optimal (Figure 1). Offspring are reared for an assessment of postnatal functional development as described above and for reproductive maturity. A caesarean section is performed on half of the dams one day prior to parturition for the evaluation of *in utero* survival and fetal weight as well as external, visceral and skeletal morphology. Alternatively, the animals are treated during organogenesis only and a caesarean section with examinations as above is performed on all dams. This approach means that the assessment of postnatal functions will have to be done in a separate study and, thus, it will demand more resources.

The design of the study for embryo-fetal development in rabbits involves the treatment of the females during days 6–18 of gestation followed by caesarean section one or two days prior to parturition, i.e. on day 28–30 of gestation. As for the rat, fetuses are examined for effects on survival, body weight and external, visceral and skeletal morphology. The strategy of developmental toxicity testing is thus based on the identification of possible developmental disturbances in initially performed studies and whether these

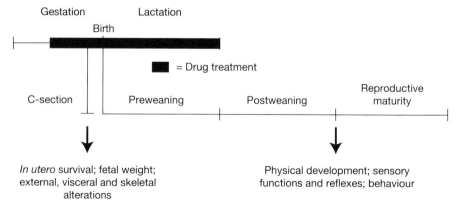

Figure 1. Design of the developmental toxicity study in the rat.

disturbances are critical to the safety assessment. When there is an effect of concern, further studies may be needed to explore the dose–response relationship, critical periods of exposure or mechanisms of action (Lumley, 1991).

BIOLOGICAL FACTORS INFLUENCING SENSITIVITY AND PREDICTIVITY

There are several factors which need to be taken into account when assessing the predictive value of teratogenicity testing in laboratory animals (Fraser, 1977). Differences between laboratory animals and humans as regards (1) pharmacokinetics, (2) gestational development sequence, (3) susceptibility at the cell, tissue or organ level, and (4) placental barrier must be considered.

Information on drug exposure and metabolite patterns in the pregnant animal and on the penetration of compound to the placental compartment is particularly important in the assessment of developmental toxicity in rats and rabbits and any other species used for developmental toxicity testing. Without this information, the results from the embryo-fetal studies cannot be adequately interpreted and assessed and difficulties will arise when the product is to be labelled as regards its effects in pregnancy and on the developing organism. In order to ensure that sufficient exposure levels are attained during all critical periods of development, and also as an assessment of the suitability of the species, some information on exposure levels and metabolite pattern should be sought prior to the conduct of the study. Although this strategy has rarely been followed in the past, it is anticipated that the recommendations given in the new international guideline should promote the performance of these basic studies.

A seemingly major problem with the rat and the rabbit as models for humans is that organogenesis in these animals occupies approximately two-thirds of the time of gestation, whereas human organogenesis takes place during about a quarter of the total gestational period. The fetal period is therefore markedly longer in humans relative to the rat and rabbit. The fact that embryos of rodent species are relatively immature at any given stage of gestation compared with the human embryo may have significant consequences when interpreting the results of developmental toxicity studies. From this perspective, non-human primates would be a much better choice than either the rat or the rabbit. However, ethical considerations as well as poor availability make the routine use of non-human primates less attractive. The limited number of animals that could be used per dose group would reduce the sensitivity of the test and the investigator would still be faced with problems of interpretation. However, whether the small treatment groups or other factors are responsible for the observed lower sensitivity in non-human primates (see below) is at present unknown.

PREDICTIVE VALUE – DATA FROM THE LITERATURE

The assumption that well designed animal studies can provide relevant information regarding risk for developmental effects in humans can only be supported by careful analysis of experimental studies in several species and appropriate human data. Schardein and co-workers (1985) analysed the ability of various species to identify 15 putative human teratogens, some of which represented pharmacological classes of compounds such as androgenic hormones, anticancer antimetabolites, anticancer alkylating agents, anticonvulsants, antithyroid agents and coumarin anticoagulants. With one exception, the coumarin anticoagulant drugs, all human teratogens had been identified by studies in one or more laboratory animals. With regard to the type of malformations induced in animals and humans, the survey indicated that the responses in the mouse and the rat were more similar to the human response than those in other species. However, the mouse and rat also showed the greatest number of nonconcordant responses (Schardein *et al.*, 1985). It may be questioned whether adequate predictivity also includes that the animal response must equal that in humans. Effects such as reduced litter size and pup viability may be good indicators of potential hazards, as was shown for thalidomide in the mouse and rat (Palmer, 1976).

In a review by the US Food and Drug Administration (Frankos, 1985), it was shown that, of 38 compounds with suspected or established birth defects in humans, all but one showed a positive finding in at least one animal species (Table 1). The mouse, rat and rabbit were able to identify 85, 80 and 60%, respectively, of these potential human teratogens. Only 30% of the compounds were positive in the non-human primate. A closer analysis of the

Table 1. Sensitivity and predictivity of animal developmental toxicity studies.

Birth defects reported in humans	
Number of compounds investigated	38
Malformations in at least one laboratory species	37
Malformations in more than one laboratory species	29
No birth defects reported in humans	
Number of compounds investigated	165
Nonteratogenic in at least one other species	130
Nonteratogenic in more than one other species	84
Nonteratogenic in all other species tested	47

Source: Adapted from Frankos, 1985.

data would be needed in order to discard the non-human primate as a suitable species for the detection of potential human teratogens. However, the review strongly suggests that studies in the non-human primate, with similar reproductive physiology to humans, may not always be sensitive enough.

The same review (Frankos, 1985) also addressed the specificity of the animal studies, i.e. to what extent there is a concordance between negative outcome in humans and negative results in animals. Although the results of this analysis, encompassing altogether 165 compounds, are far from encouraging (there was concordance in 35, 50, 70 and 80% of the cases in mice, rats, rabbits and monkeys, respectively), the comparison may in several respects be misleading. First, the information regarding potential teratogenicity in humans is not of sufficient quality to conclude firmly that these compounds are not teratogenic in humans; i.e. the number of exposed pregnant women and extent of exposure during pregnancy are not well documented. Secondly, and more importantly, exposure levels in a large proportion of the animal studies were most likely many times higher than those occurring in man, the recommendation being that the high dose level in the embryo-fetal toxicity study should induce some level of observable maternal toxicity. Therefore, if exposure levels had been considered, the outcome of the analysis would most likely have been totally different.

From the available literature it is reasonable to conclude that present testing strategies have the sensitivity to detect potential human teratogens. The high number of apparently 'false' positive results is a major problem associated with the strategies. In the absence of good clinical follow-up and adequate population monitoring of drug use during pregnancy, the rigorous pregnancy labelling which occurs as a result of the animal findings may persist over decades. As a consequence, pregnant women or women of childbearing potential may be denied therapies; this could result in significant negative health implications. Better knowledge of mechanisms of teratogenicity and increased awareness of exposure–response relationships might increase the predictivity of preclinical animal testing and reduce the number of 'false' positives. However, unless there is a concomitant effort, on a national or regional basis, to collect data on drug use during pregnancy, the information given to prescribing physicians and women will continue to be unclear and, in many instances, irrelevant.

REFERENCES

Frankos, V.H. (1985). FDA perspectives on the use of teratology data for human risk assessment. *Fundam Appl Toxicol* **5**, 615–625.
Fraser, F.C. (1977). Relation of animal studies to the problem in man. In: Wilson, J.G. and Fraser F.C. (Eds), *Handbook of Teratology. Vol. 1. General Principles and Etiology*. Plenum, New York, pp. 75–96.

ICH (International Conference on Harmonization of Technical Requirements for the Registration of Pharmaceuticals for Human Use) (1993). ICH Harmonized Tripartite Guideline; Detection of Toxicity to Reproduction for Medicinal Products. In: D'Arcy, P.F. and Harron D.W.G. (Eds), *Proceedings of the Second International Conference on Harmonization*. W & G Baird Ltd, Belfast, pp. 557–578.

Lumley, C.E. (1991). Proposal for international guidelines for reproductive and developmental toxicity testing for pharmaceuticals. *Adverse Drug React Toxicol Rev* **10**, 143–153.

Palmer, A. (1976). Assessment of current test procedures. *Environ Health Perspect* **18**, 97–104.

Schardein, J.L., Schwetz, B.A. and Kenel, M.F. (1985). Species sensitivities and prediction of teratogenic potential. *Environ Health Perspect* **61**, 55–67.

Schmid, B. (1987). Old and new concepts in teratogenicity testing. *Trends Pharmacol Sci* **8**, 133–138.

US Food and Drug Administration (USFDA) (1966). *Guidelines for Reproduction Studies for Safety Evaluation of Drug for Human Use.*

Epilepsy and Pregnancy
Edited by T. Tomson, L. Gram, M. Sillanpää and S.I. Johannessen
© 1997 Wrightson Biomedical Publishing Ltd

3

Mechanisms of Teratogenesis of Antiepileptic Drugs

BENGT R. DANIELSSON

Astra Safety Assessment, Södertälje, and Department of Pharmaceutical Biosciences, Uppsala University, Uppsala, Sweden

INTRODUCTION

The widely used antiepileptic drugs (AEDs) phenytoin (PHT), carbamazepine (CBZ), and valproic acid (VPA) have all been associated with an increased risk for birth defects in human pregnancy. *In utero* exposure to PHT and CBZ has resulted in a similar pattern of minor defects, such as midfacial and distal digital hypoplasia (Hanson, 1986; Jones *et al.*, 1989). An association between postnatal developmental delay and growth deficiency and with more severe defects such as orofacial clefts, cardiac defects and microcephaly has been established for PHT (Hanson, 1986) and proposed for CBZ (microcephaly: Jones *et al.*, 1989). Carbamazepine is teratogenic in rodents, and PTH has shown teratogenicity in mice, rats, rabbits, cats and monkeys. Using animal models it has been possible to recreate all the structural defects as well as growth and developmental retardation observed in children exposed to PHT *in utero* (Finnell and Dansky, 1991). The pattern of malformations related to VPA exposure is distinctly different from that of PHT and CBZ in both human and animal studies (Lindhout, 1993). Mechanistic studies on VPA-induced teratogenesis are therefore presented in Chapter 4 which focuses on VPA-induced neural tube defects.

The different malformation pattern between PHT and VPA together with the fact that it is possible to induce the same type of defects as observed in man in nonepileptic animals, suggest that it is the AED and not the maternal disease (or seizures) which is the major teratogenic factor. This proposal is supported by a study in inbred mice with spontaneous seizures (Finnell and Chernoff, 1982). In mice with seizures that were left untreated and which therefore had several seizures per day throughout pregnancy, the dams produced normal healthy offspring. As the dams were placed on increasing

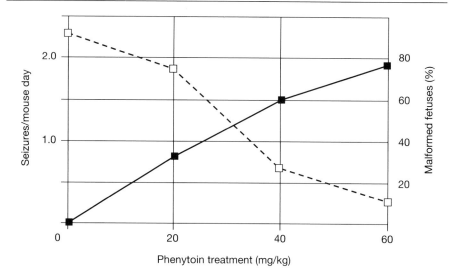

Figure 1. Effect of phenytoin on seizures (□) and malformations (■) in an inbred strain of mice (C 57 Bl/6J qk/qk). (Adapted, with permission, from Finnell and Chernhoff, 1982.)

dosages of PHT, the frequency of seizures decreased, while the incidence of malformations increased in conjunction with maternal plasma phenytoin concentration (see Figure 1). Overall, PHT has been investigated extensively in experimental studies, while mechanistic studies of CBZ and most other AEDs (with the exception of VPA) are very few (Finnell and Dansky, 1991). However, in view of the similarities in malformation pattern between PHT and CBZ (and some other AEDs such as ethotoin, and trimethadion), it is not unreasonable to assume a common mechanism for induction of malformations for these drugs. Phenytoin may thus serve as a prototype for other AEDs with similar pharmacological and teratogenic properties.

MECHANISMS FOR PHENYTOIN-INDUCED TERATOGENESIS

Several mechanisms underlying PHT teratogenicity have been proposed, including disturbances in folate metabolism (Monie *et al.*, 1961; Wilson and Fradkin, 1967), and bioactivation of PHT to a reactive toxic intermediate (epoxide) by cytochrome P-450 (Martz *et al.*, 1977; Harbison *et al.*, 1977). An alternative bioactivating pathway for the induction of malformations has been proposed involving the co-oxidation of PHT to free radical intermediates centred in the hydantoin nucleus (Wells and Vo, 1989).

A more recent theory suggests that PHT teratogenicity is mainly initiated by adverse pharmacological action on the embryonic heart during a restricted sensitive stage, resulting in embryonic hypoxia/ischaemia (Danielsson *et al.*, 1992). Maternal haemodynamic alterations may contribute to the embryonic hypoxia, but these alterations are not of such a magnitude that they alone can explain observed hypoxia-related malformations. The embryonic hypoxia/ischaemia results in vascular disruption, haemorrhage and tissue necrosis of affected embryonic/fetal tissues (Danielson *et al.*, 1992). The tissue necrosis, manifested as malformations in the fetus at term, may be a direct consequence of the hypoxia and/or generation of reactive oxygen species (ROS) at reperfusion in the same way as generation of ROS has been associated with tissue damage during reperfusion of the ischaemic heart (after myocardial infarction), and in CNS after stroke (Gutteridge, 1993; McCord, 1993).

In the following, the folate, the bioactivation and the hypoxia/reoxygenation theories will be presented and discussed. Most attention will be paid to the new hypoxia/reoxygenation hypothesis, since this theory offers an explanation for the pattern of PHT-induced malformations, and the duration of the susceptible period, as well as why other AEDs with similar pharmacological effects to PHT have been associated with similar malformations. The discussion will focus on the bioactivation hypothesis in relation to the hypoxia/reoxygenation hypothesis.

Disturbance in folate metabolism

The oldest explanation for PHT-induced teratogenesis is a disturbance in folate metabolism (Massey, 1966; Gibson and Becker, 1968; Netzloff *et al.*, 1979; Hansen and Billings, 1985). Human case-reports suggested comparable malformations in children exposed to PHT *in utero* as those in offspring of mothers treated with folinic acid antagonists, such as aminopterin and methotrexate (Thiersch, 1952; Goetsch, 1962; Milunsky *et al.*, 1968). In experimental studies, animals fed diets that were deficient in folate or a diet that contained folate antagonists showed an increased incidence of orofacial clefts and other defects (Wilson and Fradkin, 1967; Monie *et al.*, 1961). However, in studies trying to modify the teratogenicity of PHT by supplementation of various amounts of folate, folate conferred no protection against teratogenic effects. Instead, supplementation of moderate to high concentrations of folate potentiated the teratogenic effects (Schardein *et al.*, 1973). This result was confirmed in a study in another species (Mercier-Parot and Tuchmann-Duplessis, 1974). Therefore it is unclear how alterations in folate metabolism secondary to maternal PHT therapy can result in an increased incidence of malformations.

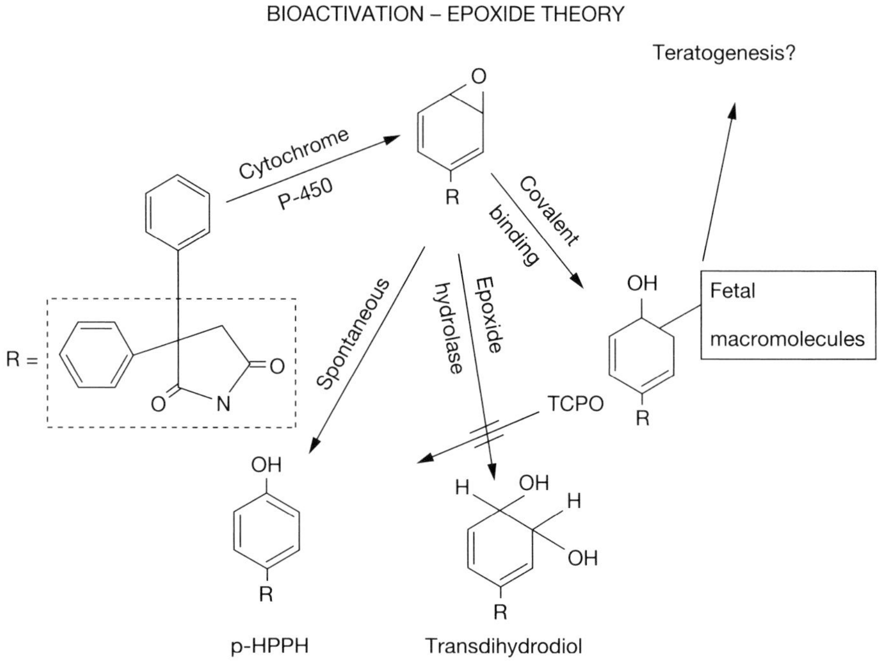

BIOACTIVATION – EPOXIDE THEORY

Figure 2. Proposed epoxide mechanism for phenytoin-induced teratogenesis. Pretreatment with trichloropropene oxide (TCPO), an inhibitor of epoxide hydrolase, increases the teratogenicity of phenytoin. (Reproduced, with permission, from Blake and Martz, 1980.)

Bioactivation of phenytoin to reactive intermediates

The most favoured theory proposes bioactivation of PHT to a toxic reactive metabolite. One school holds that the source of the teratogenicity of PHT is an arene oxide metabolite (epoxide) produced enzymatically in the maternal liver during the bioactivation of PHT by cytochrome P-450 (see Figure 2), which is capable of binding covalently to nucleic acids in embryonic tissues (Martz et al., 1977; Blake and Martz, 1980). Arene oxides, in general, are short-lived and highly reactive, and when the rate of bioactivation exceeds the detoxification capacity of the organism, the electrophilic centre of the molecule is capable of binding covalently to nucleophilic sites in embryonic macromolecules. It has been suggested that the formation of such arene oxides may be a common mechanism for certain AEDs' (PHT, CBZ and phenobarbitone) teratogenicity. It has also been proposed that interactions may occur between different AEDs as regards induction/detoxification of these reactive epoxides, which may be of importance in explaining why

BIOACTIVATION – FREE RADICAL INTERMEDIATE

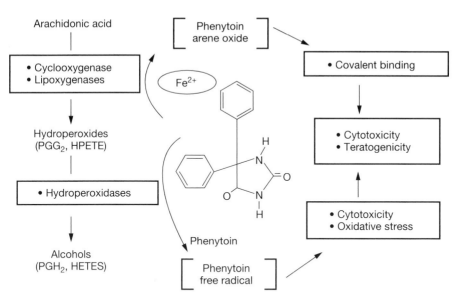

Figure 3. Postulated mechanisms of phenytoin bioactivation within the embryo by cyclo-oxygenase and lipo-oxygenases in relation to phenytoin teratogenicity. (Reproduced, with permission, from Winn and Wells, 1995.)

combination therapy with these AEDs has been associated with an increased risk for human malformations (Lindhout *et al.*, 1982; Lindhout, 1993).

An alternative bioactivating pathway involves the co-oxidation of PHT to free radical intermediates centred in the hydantoin nucleus of the PHT molecule by the enzyme prostaglandin synthetase (Kubow and Wells, 1986; Wells and Vo, 1989). It is proposed that such free radical intermediates of PHT (see Figure 3) may result in oxidative stress, initiate lipid peroxidation and/or bind covalently to DNA (Wells and Vo, 1989). Wells and colleagues have performed several studies giving evidence for the involvement of oxidative stress in PHT-teratogenesis, such as enhancement of PHT teratogenicity, inhibition of glutathione (GSH) peroxidase or GSH reductase and reduction of PHT teratogenicity by antioxidants (e.g. vitamin E), a free radical spinning agent, or the iron chelator desferoxamine (Yu and Wells, 1995). It has also been shown that mouse and rat embryos during the susceptible period for PHT teratogenesis have low activities of the endogenous antioxidants such as GSH reductase, catalase and superoxide dismutase (SOD). Addition of SOD to embryos cultured *in vitro* in a medium containing teratogenic concentrations of PHT substantially increased embryonic

SOD activity and reduced PHT-initiated embryo toxicity (Winn and Wells, 1995). In view of these findings, it is proposed that PHT teratogenesis occurs via reactive oxygen species (ROS) production secondary to bioactivation of PHT by embryonic peroxidases, (e.g. prostaglandin synthetase) in embryonic tissues (Yu and Wells, 1995).

Hypoxia/reoxygenation hypothesis

As mentioned previously, this theory suggests that PHT teratogenicity is mediated via pharmacologically induced fetal hypoxia followed by reoxygenation and generation of ROS in embryonic tissues. The role of ROS is well established in ischaemia/reperfusion damage in adult tissues after myocardial infarct and stroke. In support of the hypoxia hypothesis, the malformations induced by phenytoin are almost identical and preceded by the same early pathological changes (oedema, vascular disruption, haemorrhage and, finally, tissue necrosis) during the same stage of pregnancy as can be observed after temporary clamping of uterine vessels. Short clamping periods (30 minutes) and low teratogenic doses of PHT at the same stage of gestation in animal studies induce mainly distal digital hypoplasia, while longer clamping periods (45–90 minutes) and higher PHT doses induce more severe malformations (e.g. central nervous system (CNS) defects and severe limb amputation defects) (clamping: Leist and Grauwiler, 1974; Webster *et al.*, 1987; phenytoin: Danielson *et al.*, 1992). Furthermore, maternal hyperoxia has been shown to reduce greatly the incidence of PHT-induced malformations (Millicovsky and Johnston, 1981).

Phenytoin exerts pharmacological effects on sodium (Na^+), calcium (Ca^{++}) and potassium (K^+) channels resulting in stabilizing effects on excitable membranes of neurons and cardiac myocytes (Rall and Schleifer, 1990). These pharmacological properties explain why PHT is an effective anticonvulsant and also why PHT has been shown to be an effective drug for the treatment of ventricular arrhythmias. However, these properties may also explain PHT's capacity to induce haemodynamic alterations and severe episodes of hypoxia in the embryo/fetus. Vasodilating Ca^{++} antagonists like nifedipine, felodipine and nicardipine have all induced decreased uteroplacental blood flow and embryonic hypoxia secondary to maternal hypotension and a diversion of blood flow from the pregnant uterus to peripheral vascular beds (Ducsay *et al.*, 1987; Lirette *et al.*, 1987; Harake *et al.*, 1987; Lundgren *et al.*, 1992). These drugs have also induced hypoxia-related malformations, such as distal digital hypoplasia in animal studies (Danielsson and Webster, 1997). The Ca^{++} antagonizing properties of PHT may explain the decreased maternal blood pressure and heart rate after a teratogenic dose of PHT in pregnant animals (Watkinson and Millicovsky, 1983; Danielson *et al.*, 1992).

Table 1. Adverse effects of phenytoin (expressed as a percentage of affected embryos in relation to all embryos exposed to a certain concentration) in two strains of mouse embryo (A/J and C 57 Bl/6J). The embryos were cultured in medium containing 80% rat serum. A concentration-dependent increase in arrhythmias and cardiac arrest is observed in both mouse strains, but is more pronounced in the A/J mouse embryos.

Concentration phenytoin (μM)	C 57 Bl/6J		A/J	
	Arrhythmias	Cardiac arrest	Arrhythmias	Cardiac arrest
0	0	0	0	0
100	0	0	67	0
150	18	0	57	0
200	13	0	50	0
300	69	56	100	100
400	89	67	–	–

Source: Adapted with permission, from Danielsson *et al.*, 1997.

Phenytoin's capacity to delay K^+ currents (class III antiarrhythmic activity) during action potentials (Yaari *et al.*, 1986) may be of even greater importance in explaining its teratogenicity. Recent experimental studies using *in vitro* embryo cultures have shown that the embryonic/fetal heart during a restricted period is extremely susceptible to the pharmacological action of drugs showing an inhibitory action on K^+ channels. In the rat, the susceptibility for class III antiarrhythmics embryonic/fetal adverse effects started on gestational day 10, when the embryonic heart starts bearing, and ended on day 15 (Webster *et al.*, 1996). Severe embryonic/fetal bradycardia, temporary arrhythmia and cardiac arrest occur at dose levels which were far from causing cardiodepressive or any other signs of adverse effects in the mothers during this period (Ban *et al.*, 1992; Abrahamsson *et al.*, 1994; Spence *et al.*, 1994; Webster *et al.*, 1996). This type of compound has also induced hypoxia-related malformations, such as distal digital defects and orofacial clefts, which were preceded by oedema, haemorrhage, and necrosis (Danielsson, 1993; Webster *et al.*, 1996). Interestingly, PHT has been shown to affect the embryonic heart in exactly the same way as the above-mentioned class III antiarrhythmics. In a concentration-dependent manner PHT caused embryonic bradycardia, arrhythmias and cardiac arrest in mouse as well as rat embryos cultured *in vitro* (see Table 1 and Figure 4) during the sensitive period for induction of malformations in these species (Danielsson *et al.*, 1997). The effects were reversible, and when culture medium containing PHT was replaced with fresh medium (with no PHT) the embryonic heart rate returned to baseline values, also in embryos showing temporary/permanent arrest. The concentrations affecting the embryonic heart were comparable with those associated with PHT-induced teratogenicity in human pregnancy (Gaily, 1990) and animals (Danielsson *et al.*, 1995).

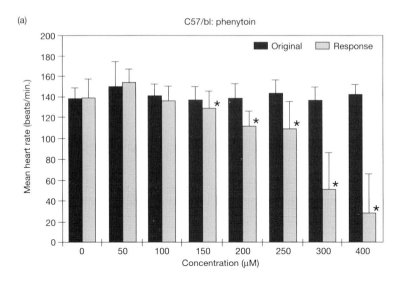

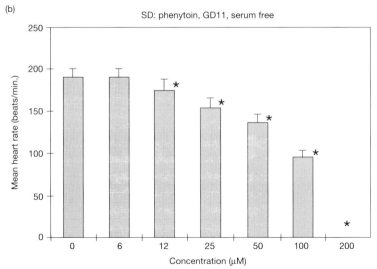

Figure 4. (a) Effects of different concentrations of phenytoin on the heart rate in day 10 C 57/Bl embryos cultured *in vitro* in medium containing 80% rat serum. Original heart rate (beats/min before addition of phenytoin) is compared with heart rate after addition of phenytoin (mean values of three measurements 30, 60, and 90 minutes after addition of phenytoin). (b) Effects of different concentrations of phenytoin on the heart rate in day 11 Sprague-Dawley rat embryos cultured in serum-free medium. This procedure makes it easier to compare concentrations when effects are obtained in this *in vitro* model with free plasma concentrations associated with malformations in human and animal studies. (Reproduced, with permission, from Danielsson *et al.*, 1997.)

Phenytoin may also cause haemodynamic alterations on the maternal side. Hypotension may occur at high therapeutic doses in humans (Bigger and Hoffman, 1980), and has also been seen in animals. A teratogenic dose in the rabbit resulting in similar free plasma concentrations (Danielsson *et al.*, 1995) as have been associated with the same type of defect in the human fetus (Gaily, 1990) caused a mild decrease in maternal blood pressure (15%) and heart rate (15%), resulting in a decrease in pO_2 of 15% (Danielson *et al.*, 1992). These maternal haemodynamic effects of PHT are relatively mild compared with the effects of a vasodilating Ca^{++} antagonist, causing identical distal digital defects as phenytoin during the same stage of gestation (days 14–16) in rabbits (Danielsson *et al.*, 1989, 1990, 1992). The vasodilator induced a marked decrease in maternal blood pressure (30%) and a drastic decrease in uteroplacental blood flow (40–50%) secondary to the hypotension and a diversion of blood flow from the pregnant uterus to peripheral vascular beds (Lundgren *et al.*, 1992) at a dose level which induced mild phalangeal hypoplasia (Danielsson *et al.*, 1989). Despite this, the phalangeal defects (and thus most likely also the fetal hypoxia) after administration of the vasodilator was much less pronounced than the phalangeal defects of PHT occurring at slight maternal haemodynamic alterations. These data strongly indicated a pharmacological effect of PHT on the fetal side, besides the mild effect on the maternal side, as explanation of observed hypoxia-related pathological changes preceding the malformations (Danielsson *et al.*, 1992).

The maternal haemodynamic alterations of PHT may, however, significantly contribute in aggravating the embryonic hypoxia induced by a direct effect on the embryonic heart by PHT. It is well known from clinical studies that the embryonic/fetal heart rate decreases dramatically under maternally mediated hypoxic conditions, e.g. decreased uteroplacental blood flow secondary to pharmacologically induced decreased maternal heart rate and/or hypotension (Spinnato *et al.*, 1986). Similar results have been shown in animal experimental studies (Chernhoff and Grabowski, 1971; Skilman *et al.*, 1985). Maternal hypoxia also results in vasoconstriction of uterine placental vessels, further compromising oxygen supply to the embryo (de Moraes *et al.*, 1995). In addition, during hypoxic conditions, the adult heart has been shown to be much more susceptible to reacting with arrhythmias than under normoxia when exposed to drugs acting on Na^+ channels, such as PHT (Bigger and Hoffman, 1980). If the same is true for the embryonic heart this may be an aggravating factor for induction of arrhythmias mediated via haemodynamic alterations in the mother.

The above implies that the embryo might have a higher risk for hypoxia-mediated malformations if PHT also induces negative haemodynamic alterations on the maternal side, in addition to the direct effects on the embryonic/fetal heart. This also indicates that the embryonic hypoxia (and

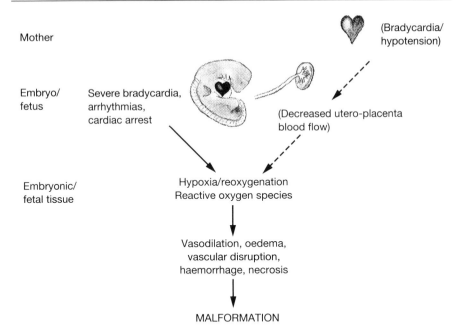

Figure 5. Hypoxia–reoxygenation as the underlying mechanism of phenytoin teratogenicity. Phenytoin induces concentration-dependent embryonic bradycardia and arrhythmia resulting in hypoxia and free oxygen radical damage at reoxygenation. Maternal haemodynamic alterations (bradycardia/hypotension) may contribute to the embryonic hypoxia. The malformations are preceded by specific histopathological changes (vasodilation, oedema, vascular disruption, haemorrhage and, finally, necrosis) in embryonic tissues. (Reproduced with permission, from Danielsson *et al.*, 1997.)

thus also the risk for hypoxia-related malformations) is greater in the *in vivo* situation than in the whole-embryo culture model. Despite this, the 'free' PHT concentrations inducing significant adverse effects on the embryonic heart *in vitro* were very close to those associated with malformations in humans and *in vivo* animal studies (Danielsson *et al.*, 1995). This result further emphasizes that the direct effect on the embryonic heart is the main factor for initiation of PHT teratogenesis (Figure 5). However, the different genetic sensitivity for PHT-induced malformations may partly be a consequence of more aggravated maternal haemodynamic alterations (resulting in a more severe embryonic hypoxia in sensitive strains/species/individuals). In a study by Watkinson and Millicovsky (1983), the same dose of PHT caused a drastic decrease in maternal heart rate in A/J strain, while the effects in C 57 Bl/6J strain were much less pronounced. The increased susceptibility of the A/J strain to PHT teratogenicity in relation to the C 57 Bl/6J strain has in other studies been shown *not* to be correlated to maternal kinetics (Roberts *et al.*, 1991), production of arene-oxide metabolites or other maternally generated metabolites (Hansen and Hodes, 1983).

DISCUSSION

This section will discuss the bioactivation hypothesis in relation to the hypothesis suggesting that the teratogenicity of PHT (and AED with similar pharmacological effects) is secondary to pharmacologically induced embryonic hypoxia, followed by generation of ROS at reoxygenation in embryonic tissues. Several studies have been conducted suggesting that PHT is the primary teratogen and not one of its metabolites. Harbison and Becker (1970, 1971) showed that phenobarbital treatment (leading to increased formation of metabolites and reduced concentrations of PHT) reduced the incidence of malformations while SKF 525 pretreatment (resulting in lesser generation of metabolites and higher PHT concentrations in the mother and fetus) increased the incidence of fetal defects. This research also showed that, at doses of PHT which induced malformations, none of the major metabolites induced birth defects despite administration of two to four times the equimolar equivalent of a teratogenic dose of PHT (Harbison and Becker, 1974). Furthermore, as mentioned previously, the increased sensitivity of the A/J strain to PHT teratogenicity, in relation to the C 57 Bl strain, has been shown not to be correlated to maternal kinetics (Roberts *et al.*, 1991) or production of arene-oxide metabolites or other maternally generated metabolites (Hansen and Hodes, 1983).

There is also other specific evidence against the hypothesis of bioactivation of PHT to an arene oxide (epoxide). It is unlikely that highly reactive PHT metabolites (generated in the maternal liver by cytochrome P-450) pass the placenta. In view of the very low content and activity of cytochrome P-450 in the embryo during the sensitive days for PHT-induced malformations (Winn and Wells, 1995), a bioactivation of PHT to such a metabolite within the embryo is also unlikely. Another argument against this hypothesis is that ethotoin has been associated in several cases in human pregnancies with similar malformations (including distal digital defects) to PHT. Ethotoin, like PHT, is a hydantoin and has similar pharmacological properties. Unlike PHT ethotoin is not metabolized through an epoxide metabolite. The presence of clinical features associated with PHT by ethotoin therefore suggests that epoxide metabolites are not the causative agents in PHT-induced teratogenesis (Finnell and DiLiberti, 1983). The fact that several chemically different cardiovascular active compounds (with capacity to cause embryonic hypoxia), such as vasodilators and class III antiarrhythmics, all induce the same types of malformations, preceded by the same pathological changes as

PHT, also strongly indicates that bioactivation is not a major factor in PHT-induced teratogenesis.

However, some results supporting the idea of bioactivation of PHT to reactive intermediates may not contradict the hypoxia theory. One example is the fact that inhibition of one of the alternative metabolic pathways for PHT (mixed function oxide enzymes by the inhibitor SKF 525A) results in enhancement of the incidence of PHT-induced malformations, an increase in plasma PHT concentrations and a decrease in its elimination. This has been interpreted as an opportunity for more free drug to oxidize, which could markedly elevate the concentration of arene oxides produced (Wells and Harbison, 1980). However, the increased plasma concentrations of PHT may cause more severe embryonic hypoxia secondary to aggravated embryonic/maternal cardiovascular pharmacological effects, thereby supporting the hypoxia theory. Other such examples are studies showing decreased teratogenicity of PHT after co-administration of PHT and antioxidants, glutathione or radical spin-trapping agents. All these agents have the capacity to reduce the tissue binding of reactive metabolites of PHT (Finnell and Dansky, 1991), or reactive species generated by oxidative stress reactions (e.g. lipid peroxidation) proposed to be initiated by the bioactivation of PHT to a free radical intermediate centred in the hydantoin nucleus by prostaglandin synthetase (Yu and Wells, 1995).

Interestingly, transient hypoxia followed by reoxygenation has also been shown to generate reactive oxygen species. Shortly after reoxygenation, after two transient hypoxia periods (each 30 minutes) on gestational day 14 *in vitro* cultured rat embryos, superoxide anion radicals were detected in the limb buds. The transient hypoxia periods resulted in distal digital hypoplasia, which was preceded by vascular disruption and haemorrhage (Fantel *et al.*, 1992; Barber *et al.*, 1993). As mentioned previously, PHT (Danielson *et al.*, 1992), the class III antiarrhythmic agents almokalant and dofetilide (Webster *et al.*, 1996) and clamping of uterine vessels (Leist and Grauwiler, 1974) all induce the same defects *in vivo* at the same gestational stage. In all cases the defects were preceded by vascular disruption and haemorrhage. Temporary embryonic/fetal hypoxia of longer duration during other stages of pregnancy may cause other types of malformation, such as cleft palate, CNS, cardiac and urogenital malformations and more severe amputation defects of the limbs (in all cases preceded by haemorrhage) as shown in uterine vessel clamping studies (Brent and Franklin, 1960; Franklin and Brent, 1964; Leist and Grauwiler, 1974; Webster *et al.*, 1987). All these malformations have been associated with PHT exposure during pregnancy in humans and in animal studies (review Dansky and Finnell, 1991; Finnell and Dansky, 1991).

The increased sensitivity of specific embryonic tissues to transient hypoxia has been correlated with the increased generation of superoxide anion radicals, due to low activities of superoxide dismutase (SOD) in sensitive tissue. In insensitive tissue, there was higher SOD activity and lower generation of superoxide anion radicals than in the teratogenically sensitive tissue (Fantel *et al.*, 1995). These findings, together with the fact that the hypoxia/ischaemia is more pronounced in the distal parts of the body (e.g. distal phalanges and tip of the nose), may be of importance in explaining the pattern of malformation induced by PHT and other compounds causing hypoxia. The conditions for generation of superoxide radicals (and even more toxic ROS) after hypoxia/reoxygenation as well as the content and activities of endogenous antioxidants (SOD, GSH etc.) may change during development. This may explain why a certain embry-onic/fetal tissue is not teratogenically sensitive during the whole suscepti-ble period. In contrast to other proposed mechanisms, pharmacologically mediated embryonic hypoxia followed by reoxygenation may explain the pattern of PHT-induced malformations as well as the susceptible period. Also, in contrast to other hypotheses, the hypoxia theory may explain other manifestations after *in utero* exposure to PHT, such as growth and mental retardation. In addition, this hypothesis may explain why PHT and other cardioactive antiepileptics with stabilizing effects on excitable membranes have been associated with a similar pattern of malformations and why polytherapy with such drugs seems to increase the risk for malformations (Lindhout, 1993).

A comment in relation to the hypoxia-reoxygenation theory is that a genetic susceptibility to the cardiodepressive effect of PHT may be of impor-tance in explaining species/strain/individual differences in PHT teratogenic-ity. Future comparative studies between different strains/species concerning (1) PHT-induction of embryonic arrhythmias, (2) PHT-induced haemody-namic alterations in the intact pregnant animal and (3) content and activities of antioxidants in embryonic tissues, may help to explain why some embryos are more sensitive to the teratogenic action of PHT than others, despite being exposed to identical plasma concentrations.

In conclusion, mechanistic studies have been very beneficial in validating the teratogenicity of selected AEDs and in providing information on pharmacokinetic parameters of importance for assessing at which plasma concentrations adverse fetal effects may occur. Animal studies are invaluable when elucidating the mechanisms of teratogenic action, since it is possible to examine, in detail, the pathogenesis of the congenital abnormality, and not only the final manifestation. Animal studies can help develop the experi-mental data to support alterations in human therapeutic practices that may be successful in limiting or reducing the adverse effects of AED therapy during pregnancy. Finally, more knowledge on the mechanisms of AED teratogenicity may contribute to the development of new AEDs without teratogenic properties.

ACKNOWLEDGEMENTS

The author gratefully acknowledges the assistance of Ms Maria Sundkvist in preparing this chapter and the financial support of CFN and MFR for mechanistic studies of teratogenesis of antiepileptic drugs.

REFERENCES

Abrahamsson, C., Palmer, M., Ljung, B. *et al.* (1994). Induction of rhythm abnormalities in the fetal rat heart. A tentative mechanism for the embryotoxic effect of class III antiarrhythmic agent almokalant. *Cardiovasc Res* **28**, 337–344.

Ban, Y., Konishi, R., Kawana, K., Nakatsuka, T. and Fujii, T. (1992). Embryonic effects of class III antiarrhythmic agent, L-691, 121 in rats. *Teratology* **45**, 462.

Barber, C.V., Carda, M.B. and Fantel, A.G. (1993). A new technique for culturing rat embryos *in vitro* between gestation day 14 and 15. *Toxicol In Vitro* **7**, 695–700.

Bigger, J.T. and Hoffman, B.F. (1980). Antiarrhythmic drugs. In: Gilman, A.G., Goodman, L.S. and Gilman, A. (Eds), *The Pharmacological Basis of Therapeutics, (6th edn)*. Macmillan, New York, pp. 761–792.

Blake, D.A. and Martz, F. (1980). Covalent binding of phenytoin metabolites in fetal tissue. In: Hassell, T.M., Johnston, M.C. and Dudley, K.H. (Eds), *Phenytoin-induced Teratology and Gingival Pathology*. Raven Press, New York, pp. 75–80.

Brent, R.L. and Franklin, J.B. (1960). Uterine vascular clamping: new procedures for the study of congenital malformations. *Science* **132**, 89–91.

Chernhoff, N. and Grabowski, C.T. (1971). Responses of the rat foetus to maternal injections of adrenalin and vasopressin. *Br J Pharmacol* **43**, 270–278.

Danielson, M.K., Danielsson, B.R.G., Marchner, H., Lundin, M., Rundqvist, E. and Reiland, S. (1992). Histopathological and hemodynamic studies supporting hypoxia and vascular disruption as explanation to phenytoin teratogenicity. *Teratology* **46**, 485–497.

Danielsson, B.R. (1993). Malformations and fetal hypoxia induced by exaggerated pharmacological effects. In: Sundvall, A., Danielsson, B.R., Hagberg, O., Lindgren, E., Sjöberg, P. and Victor, A. (Eds), *Developmental Toxicology – Preclinical and Clinical Data in Retrospect*. Tryckgruppen, Stockholm, pp. 44–57.

Danielsson, B.R. and Webster, W.S. (1997). Cardiovascular active drugs. In: Kavlock, R.J. and Daston, G. (Eds), *Drug Toxicity in Embryonic Development. Handbook of Experimental Pharmacology*. Springer-Verlag, New York, pp. 161–190.

Danielsson, B.R.G., Reiland, S., Rundqvist, E. and Danielson, M. (1989). Digital defects induced by vaso-dilating agents. Relationship to reduction in utero-placental blood flow. *Teratology* **40**, 351–357.

Danielsson, B.R.G., Reiland, S., Rundqvist, E., Danielson, M., Dencker, L. and Regård, C.-G. (1990). Histological and *in vitro* studies supporting decreased utero-placental blood flow as explanation to digital defects after administration of vasodilators. *Teratology* **41**, 185–193.

Danielsson, B.R.G., Danielson, M., Rundqvist, E. and Reiland, S. (1992). Identical phalangeal defects induced by phenytoin and nifedipine suggest fetal hypoxia and vascular disruption behind phenytoin teratogenicity. *Teratology* **45**, 247–258.

Danielsson, B.R.G., Danielson, K. and Tomson, T. (1995). Phenytoin causes phalangeal hypoxia in the rabbit fetus at clinically relevant concentrations. *Teratology* **52**, 252–259.

Danielsson, B.R., Azarbayani, F., Wisén, A.-C. and Webster, W.S. (1997). Initiation of phenytoin teratogenesis: Pharmacologically induced embryonic bradycardia and arrhythmia resulting in hypoxia and possible free radical damage at reoxygenation. *Teratology* (in press).

Dansky, V.L. and Finnell, R.H. (1991). Parental epilepsy, anticonvulsant drugs, and reproductive outcome: epidemiologic and experimental findings spanning three decades; 2: human studies. *Reprod Toxicol* **5**, 301–335.

de Moraes, S., Carvalho, J.C.A., Mathias, R.S. and Cavalcante, M.I. (1995). Reactive hypoxia-induced contraction of the isolated human umbilical artery. *Pharmacol Toxicol* **76**, 218–220.

Ducsay, C.A., Thompson, J.S., Wu, A.T. *et al.* (1987). Effects of calcium entry blocker (nicardipine) tocolysis in rhesus macaques: fetal plasma concentrations and cardiorespiratory changes. *Am J Obstet Gynecol* **157**, 1482–1486.

Fantel, A.G., Barber, C.V. and MacKler, B. (1992). Ischemia/reperfusion: a new hypothesis for the developmental toxicity of cocaine. *Teratology* **46**, 285–292.

Fantel, A.G., Person, R.E., Tumbic, R.W., Nguyen, T.D. and MacKler, B. (1995). Studies of mitochondria in oxidative embryotoxicity. *Teratology* **52**, 190–195.

Finnell, R.H. and Chernoff, G.F. (1982). Mouse feta hydantoin syndrome: effects of maternal seizures. *Epilepsia* **23**, 423–429.

Finnell, R.H. and Dansky, L.V. (1991). Parental epilepsy, anticonvulsant drugs, and reproductive outcome: epidemiologic and experimental findings spanning three decades; 1: animal studies. *Reprod Toxicol* **5**, 281–299.

Finnell, R.H. and DiLiberti J.H. (1983). Hydantoin induced teratogenesis: are some oxide intermediates really responsible? *Helv Paediatr Acta* **38**, 171–177.

Franklin, J.B. and Brent, R.L. (1964). The effect of uterine vascular clamping on the development of rat embryos three to fourteen days old. *J Morph* **115**, 273–290.

Gaily, E. (1990). Distal phalangeal hypoplasia in children with prenatal phenytoin exposure. *Am J Med Genet* **35**, 403–414.

Gibson, J.E. and Becker, B.A. (1968). Teratogenic effects of diphenylhydantoin in Swiss-Webster and A/J mice. *Proc Soc Exp Biol Med* **128**, 905–909.

Goetsch, C. (1962). An evaluation of aminopterin as an abortifacient. *Am J Obstet Gynecol* **83**, 1474–1477.

Gutteridge, J.M.C. (1993). Free radicals in disease processes. A complication of cause and consequence. *Free Rad Comm* **19**, 141–158.

Hansen, D.K. and Hodes, E. (1983). Metabolism of phenytoin in teratogenesis-susceptible and -resistant strains of mice. *Drug Metab Disp* **11**, 21–24.

Hansen, D.K. and Billings, R.E. (1985). Phenytoin teratogenicity and effects on embryonic and maternal folate metabolism. *Teratology* **31**, 363–371.

Hanson, J.W. (1986). Teratogen update: fetal hydantoin effects. *Teratology* **33**, 349–353.

Harake, B., Gilbert, R.D., Ashwal, S. and Power, G.G. (1987). Nifedipine: effects on fetal and maternal hemodynamics in pregnant sheep. *Am J Obstet Gynecol* **157**, 1003–1008.

Harbison, R.D. and Becker, B.A. (1970). Effect of phenobarbital and SKF 525A pretreatment on diphenylhydantoin teratogenicity in mice. *J Pharmacol Exp Ther* **175**, 283–288.

Harbison, R.D. and Becker, B.A. (1971). Effects of phenobarbital or SKF 525A pretreatment on diphenylhydantoin disposition in pregnant mice. *Toxicol Appl Pharmacol* **20**, 573–581.

Harbison, R.D. and Becker, B.A. (1974). Comparative embryotoxicity of diphenyl-hydantoin and some of its metabolites in mice. *Teratology* **10**, 237–241.

Harbison, R.D., MacDonald, J.S., Sweetman, B.J. and Taber, D. (1977). Proposed mechanism for diphenylhydantoin-induced teratogenesis. *Pharmacologist* **19**, 179.

Jones, K.L., Lacro, R.V., Johnson, K.A. and Adams, J. (1989). Pattern of malformations in the children of women treated with carbamazepine during pregnancy. *N Engl J Med* **320**, 1661–1666.

Kubow, S. and Wells, P.G. (1986). *In vitro* evidence for prostaglandin synthetase-catalyzed bioactivation of phenytoin to a free radical intermediate. *Pharmacologist* **28**, 195.

Leist, K.H. and Grauwiler, J. (1974). Fetal pathology in rats following uterine vessel clamping on day 14 of gestation. *Teratology* **10**, 55–68.

Lindhout, D. (1993). Antiepileptic drugs – clinical results and mechanisms. In: Sundvall, A., Danielsson, B.R., Hagber, O., Lindgren, E., Sjöberg, P. and Victor, A. (Eds), *Developmental Toxicology – Preclinical and Clinical Data in Retrospect*. Tryckgruppen, Stockholm, pp. 111–121.

Lindhout, D., Meinardi, H. and Barth, P.G. (1982). Hazards of fetal exposure to drug combinations. In: Janz, D., Dam, M., Richens, A. *et al.* (Eds), *Epilepsy, Pregnancy and the Child*. New York, Raven Press, pp. 275–281.

Lirette, M., Holbrook, R.H. and Katz, M. (1987). Cardiovascular and uterine blood flow changes during nicaripine HCl tocolysis in the rabbit. *Obstet Gynecol* **69**, 79–82.

Lundgren, Y., Yhalen, P. and Nordlander, M. (1992). Effects of felodipine on utero-placental blood flow in normotensive rabbits. *Pharmacol Toxicol* **71**, 361–364.

Martz, F., Failinger, C. and Blake, D.A. (1977). Phenytoin teratogenesis in correlation between embryopathic effect and covalent binding of putative arene oxide metabolic in gestational tissue. *J Pharmacol Exp Ther* **203**, 231–239.

Massey, K.M. (1966). Teratogenic effects of diphenylhydantoin sodium. *J Oral Ther Pharmacol* **2**, 380–385.

McCord, J.M. (1993). Human disease, free radicals and the oxidant/antioxidant balance. *Clin Biochem* **26**, 261–274.

Mercier-Parot, L. and Tuchmann-Duplessis, H. (1974). The dysmorphogenic potential of phenytoin: experimental observations. *Drugs* **8**, 340–353.

Millicovsky, G. and Johnston, M.C. (1981). Maternal hyperoxia greatly reduces the incidence of phenytoin-induced cleft lip and palate in A/J mice. *Science* **212**, 671–672.

Milunsky, A., Graef, J.W. and Gaynor, M.F. (1968). Methotrexate-induced congenital malformations. *J Pediatr* **72**, 790–795.

Monie, I.W., Armstrong, R.G. and Nelson, M.M. (1961). Hydrocephalus and other abnormalities in rat young resulting from maternal pteroylglutamic acid deficiency from the 8th to 10th days of pregnancy. *Teratology* **1**, 8.

Netzloff, M.L., Streiff, R.R., Frias, J.L. and Rennert, O.M. (1979). Folate antagonism following teratogenic exposure to diphenylhydantoin. *Teratology* **19**, 45–50.

Rall, T.W. and Schleifer, L.S. (1990). Drugs effective in the therapy of epilepsy. In: Goodman Gilman, A., Rall, T.W., Nies, A.S. and Taylor, P. (Eds), *Goodman Gilman's 'The Pharmacological Basis of Therapeutics'*. Pergamon Press, New York, pp. 436–462.

Roberts, L.G., Laborde, J.B. and Slikker, W. (1991). Phenytoin teratogenicity and midgestational pharmacokinetics in mice. *Teratology* **44**, 497–505.

Schardein, J.L., Dresner, A.J., Hentz, H.L., Petrere, J.A., Fitzgerald, J.E. and Kurtz, S.M. (1973). The modifying effect of folinic acid on diphenylhydantoin-induced teratogenicity in mice. *Toxicol Appl Pharmacol* **24**, 150–158.

Skillman, C.A., Plessinger, M.A., Woods, J.R. and Clark, K.E. (1985). Effects of graded reduction in uteroplacental blood flow in the fetal lamb. *Am J Physiol* **249**, 1098–1105.

Spence, G.S., Vetter, C. and Hoe, C.-M. (1994). Effects of the class III antiarrhythmic, dofetilide (UK-68,798) on the heart rate of midgestation rat embryos *in vitro*. *Teratology* **49**, 282–292.

Spinnato, J.A., Sibai, B.M. and Anderson, G.D. (1986). Fetal distress after hydralazine therapy for severe pregnancy-induced hypertension. *South Med J* **79**, 559–562.

Thiersch, J.B. (1952). The control of reproduction in rats with the aid of antimetabolites and early experiments with antimetabolites as abortifacient agents in man. *Acta Endocrinol* **23** (suppl 28), 37–45.

Watkinson, W.P. and Millicovsky, G. (1983). Effect of phenytoin on maternal heart rate in A/J mice: possible role in teratogenesis. *Teratology* **28**, 1–8.

Webster, W.S., Lipson, A.H. and Brown-Woodman, P.D.C. (1987). Uterine trauma and limb defects. *Teratology* **35**, 253–260.

Webster, W.S., Brown-Woodman, P.D.C., Snow, M. and Danielsson, B.R.G. (1996). Teratogenic potential of almokalant, dofetilide, and d-sotalol: drugs with potassium channel blocking activity. *Teratology* **53**, 168–175.

Wells, P.G. and Harbison, R.D. (1980). Significance of the phenytoin reactive arene oxide intermediate, its oxepin tautomer, and clinical factors modifying their roles in phenytoin-induced teratology. In: Hassel, T.M., Johnston, M.C. and Dudley, K.H. (Eds), *Phenytoin-Induced Teratology and Gingival Pathology*. Raven Press, New York, pp. 83–108.

Wells, P.G. and Vo, H.P.N. (1989). Effects of the tumor promoter 12-0-tetradecanolylphorbol-13-acetate on phenytoin-induced embryopathy in mice. *Toxicol Appl Pharmacol* **97**, 398–405.

Wilson, J.G. and Fradkin, R. (1967). Interrelations of mortality and malformations in rats. *Teratology* **7**, 57–58.

Winn, M. and Wells, P.G. (1995). Phenytoin-initiated DNA oxidation in murine embryo culture, and embryo protection by the antioxidative enzymes superoxide dismutase and catalase: evidence for reactive oxygen species-mediated DNA oxidation in the molecular mechanism of phenytoin teratogenicity. *Mol Pharmacol* **48**, 112–120.

Yaari, Y., Selzor, M.E. and Pineus, J.H. (1986). Phenytoin: mechanisms of its anticonvulsant action. *Ann Neurol* **20**, 171–184.

Yu, W.K. and Wells, P.G. (1995). Evidence for lipoxygenase-catalyzed bioactivation of phenytoin to a teratogenic reactive intermediate: *in vitro* studies using linoleic acid-dependent soybean lipoxygenase, and *in vivo* studies using pregnant CD-1 mice. *Toxicol Appl Pharmacol* **131**, 1–12.

Epilepsy and Pregnancy
Edited by T. Tomson, L. Gram, M. Sillanpää and S.I. Johannessen
© 1997 Wrightson Biomedical Publishing Ltd

4

Towards the Mechanism of Valproic Acid Induced Neural Tube Defects

HEINZ NAU

Centre of Food Sciences, Veterinary Medical University, Hannover, Germany

INTRODUCTION

Antiepileptic drug therapy with valproic acid (VPA) (2-*n*-propylpentanoic acid) has been related to teratogenicity, particularly the induction of neural tube defects in humans. Retrospective (Robert, 1988) and prospective studies (Nau *et al.*, 1981a; Jäger-Roman *et al.*, 1986; Lindhout and Schmidt, 1986) have established that exposure to VPA during early pregnancy (organo-genesis) can result in a significant incidence (1–2%) of spina bifida aperta (myeloschisis).

SPECIES DIFFERENCES

Spina bifida aperta can be produced with VPA in mice (Nau *et al.*, 1991). Administration of VPA on day 8 of gestation resulted in high rates of exencephaly, a malformation of the anterior neural tube (Nau *et al.*, 1981b; Turner *et al.*, 1990). VPA appears to induce specifically spina bifida in the human, not neural tube defects in general. We investigated whether post-erior neural tube defects can also be induced by VPA in the mouse in order to develop a practical and relevant animal model. We found that adminis-tration of three consecutive high doses of VPA on day 9 of gestation (one day after the peak sensitivity to the induction of exencephaly in this species) produced a significant rate of lumbosacral spina bifida aperta (4–6% of live fetuses after doses of 450 or 500 mg/kg). Spina bifida occulta, as demon-strated in double-stained fetal skeletons by measurement of the distance between the cartilaginous ends of the vertebral arches, was produced with high frequency at low doses (Ehlers *et al.*, 1991).

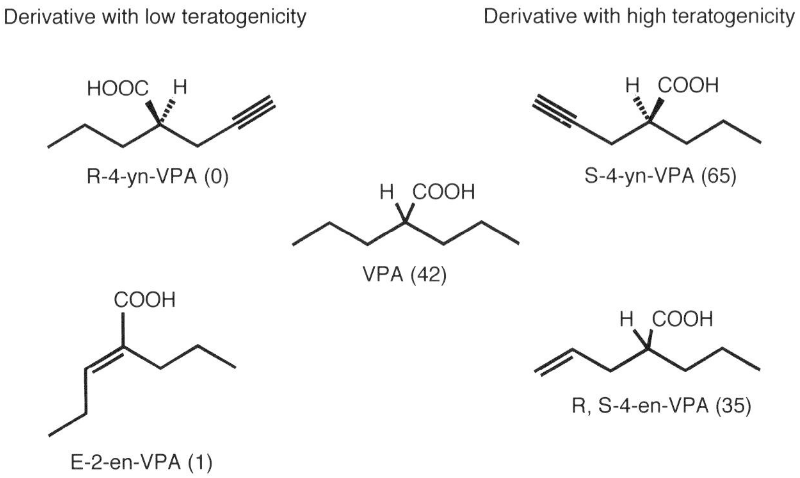

Derivative with low teratogenicity   Derivative with high teratogenicity

Figure 1. Neural tube defects in mouse offspring after treatment of the mothers with VPA and its analogues. Figures in brackets represent the percentage of exencephaly found in live fetuses on day 18 of gestation (end of term) after treatment of the dams with a single dose (3 mmol/kg b.wt; except S-4-yn-VPA 1.05 mmol/kg b.wt) of the sodium salts of the substances intraperitoneally on day 8 of gestation.

STRUCTURE–TERATOGENICITY RELATIONSHIPS

Because the parent drug molecule and not a metabolite is responsible for formation of neural tube defects in the mouse, we have investigated the teratogenic potency of a number of compounds structurally related to VPA. The aim of these studies was to determine the structural elements responsible for the teratogenic potency of this class of compounds. This should help to obtain information about the mechanism of teratogenic action of VPA and to develop alternative antiepileptic agents with low teratogenicity (Nau et al., 1991).

A strict structural requirement of expression of teratogenic effects was found (Figure 1) (Nau, 1986; Nau and Löscher, 1986). The results suggest that the following structural features are necessary to induce significant exencephaly in the mouse: (a) the α-carbon atom must be tetrahedral (sp^3 hybridization). It must be connected (b) to a free carboxyl function, (c) to a hydrogen atom, and (d) to two alkyl groups (branching on C-2 is required). Introduction (e) of a double bond between C-2 and C-3 or between C-3 and C-4 abolishes teratogenic activity. Introduction (f) of a double bond (R,S-4-en-VPA) or a triple bond (R,S-4-yn-VPA) in the 4-position results in molecules with high teratogenic activity (Nau and Löscher, 1986; Hauck and

Nau, 1989a,b; Hauck *et al.*, 1990). The anticonvulsant effect showed a much more limited dependency on the chemical structures of this class of carboxylic acids (Elmazar *et al.*, 1993).

If the two chains on C-2 differ, C-2 becomes asymmetric (binding to four different substituents), resulting in enantiomer formation. The exencephaly response was found to be highly enantioselective. The compounds with higher teratogenicity (R,S-4-yn-VPA > R,S-4-en-VPA) showed greater enantioselectivity (Hauck and Nau, 1989a; Hauck *et al.*, 1990; Andrews *et al.*, 1995). This suggests that the chiral centre on C-2 is directly involved in the process leading to neural tube defects. The nature of such a stereoselective interaction between the drug and the chiral structure within the embryo is unknown.

INTERACTION WITH EMBRYONIC FOLATE-HOMOCYSTEINE-METHIONINE METABOLISM

Periconceptional administration of multivitamins, particularly folate, was shown to reduce the recurrence risk of neural tube defects (Smithells, 1984; Laurence *et al.*, 1981; MRC Vitamin Study Research Group, 1991; Czeizel and Dudás, 1992). Antiepileptic agents such as VPA (Carl, 1986) and pheny-toin (5,5-diphenyl-2,4-imidazolidinedione) were shown to interfere with the folate metabolic pathways in the embryo (Hansen and Billings, 1985; Will *et al.*, 1985). Furthermore, folate concentrations decrease during pregnancy and treatment with antiepileptic drugs, including VPA, intensifies this effect (Hendel *et al.*, 1984). Several reports suggest that epileptic patients with malformed infants had particularly low levels of folate in their plasma (Ogawa *et al.*, 1991; Daly *et al.*, 1995). A defect of homocysteine metabolism which is interrelated with the folate pathway was found in patients with a history of offspring with neural tube defects (Steegers-Theunissen *et al.*, 1991). A mutated methylenetetrahydrofolate reductase, which forms 5-methyl-tetrahydrofolate from 5,10-methylenetetrahydrofolate, may be at the basis of these findings, because a decreased activity of this enzyme may result in low plasma folate levels, in particular 5-methyltetrahydrofolic acid, and high homocysteine concentrations (van der Put *et al.*, 1995). Taken collec-tively, these studies suggest that a genetically altered folate metabolism and/or interference with folate metabolism by antiepileptic agents may be in part responsible for the malformations observed.

We first tried to reduce the occurrence of VPA-induced exencephaly in the mouse by coadministration of folinic acid (5-formyl-tetrahydrofolic acid, 5-CHO-THF). In many cases the rate of exencephaly was significantly reduced (to 30–50% of initial rates) (Trotz *et al.*, 1987); in some cases, however, little protection was observed. These difficulties may be related to the large diurnal fluctuations of folate metabolite concentrations in the embryo (Wegner and Nau, 1991, 1992).

Teratogenic doses of VPA induced a characteristic dose-dependent alteration of embryonic folate metabolism (Wegner and Nau, 1992). The amounts of formylated folates, particularly 5-CHO-THF, decreased, while the amount of tetrahydrofolic acid (THF) increased. Comparable doses of the nonteratogenic analogue 2-en-VPA did not affect embryonic folate metabolism. The relative change in folate metabolite concentrations suggests that the interconversion between THF and 5-CHO-THF may have been inhibited by VPA. The relevant enzyme, glutamate formyltransferase, was inhibited by VPA *in vitro*; at teratogenic concentrations of VPA the activity of this enzyme was only one-third of its initial value. Furthermore, trimethoprim (Elmazar and Nau, 1993) and methotrexate (Elmazar and Nau, 1992), both inhibitors of the dihydrofolate reductase, potentiated the VPA-induced neural tube defects in mice. Collectively, these results do suggest that interference with embryonic folate metabolism may be involved in some aspects of VPA teratogenesis.

The precise molecular mechanism is unknown. It could be that the homocysteine-methionine metabolism plays a crucial role also. Homocysteine is methylated to methionine via methionine synthase using 5-methyl-tetrahydrofolate as methyl-donor. Methionine, in the form of *S*-adenosyl-methionine, is involved in numerous methylation reactions, and it may well be that VPA could directly or indirectly – via altered folate metabolism – interfere with the homocysteine–methionine pathway. We have recently obtained support in this direction by showing that methionine co-administration indeed reduced the VPA-induced spina bifida rate in mice without altering VPA kinetics (Ehlers *et al.*, 1996). Also, homocysteine increased in VPA-treated animals (Hishida *et al.*, unpublished results), reinforcing the importance of the interrelationship between the folate and homocysteine–methionine pathways.

ALTERATION OF ENDOGENOUS RETINOID LEVELS AS POSSIBLE MECHANISM OF TERATOGENESIS OF VPA AND OTHER ANTIEPILEPTIC AGENTS

Vitamin A and retinoids are thought to control many processes of embryonic development including growth, differentiation and morphogenesis. We have tested the hypothesis that the teratogenic action of some antiepileptic agents is mediated via alteration of the endogenous vitamin A-retinoid metabolism. Retinol and its oxidative metabolites, all-*trans*-, 13-*cis* and 13-*cis*-4-oxo-retinoic acid (Figure 2) were measured in the plasma of 75 infants and children treated with various antiepileptic drugs for the control of

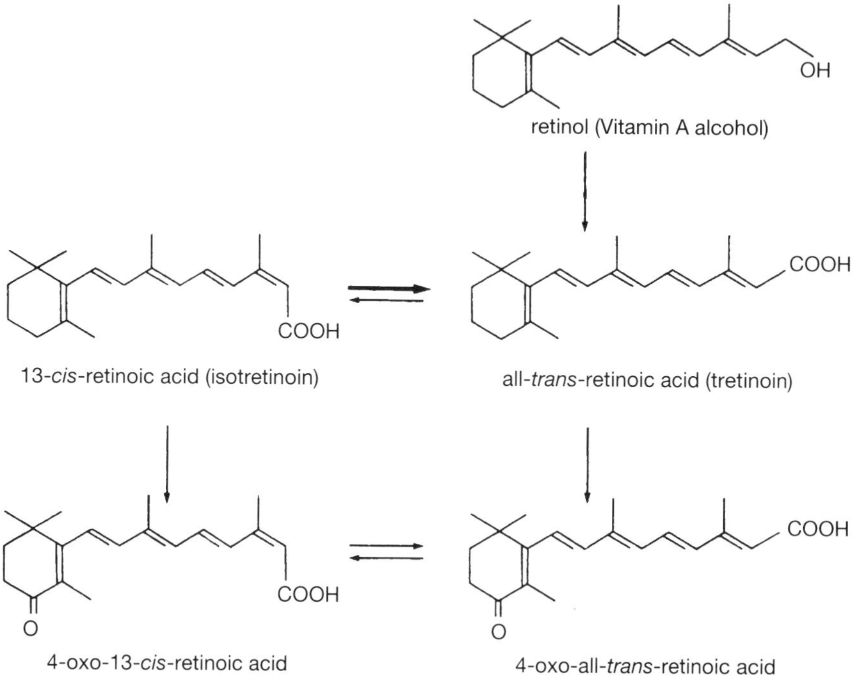

retinol (Vitamin A alcohol)

13-*cis*-retinoic acid (isotretinoin)

all-*trans*-retinoic acid (tretinoin)

4-oxo-13-*cis*-retinoic acid

4-oxo-all-*trans*-retinoic acid

Figure 2. Pattern of vitamin A metabolism discussed here. VPA may inhibit the oxidation of retinol and may also affect the further metabolism of the retinoic acid isomers; the latter pathways may be induced by other antiepileptic agents such as phenytoin, phenobarbital and carbamazepine.

seizures, and in 29 untreated controls of comparable age (Nau *et al.*, 1995). Retinol levels increased with age, while the concentrations of retinoic acid compounds did not exhibit age-dependency. Valproic acid monotherapy increased retinol levels in the young age group and a trend towards increased retinol concentrations was also observed in all other patient groups. The levels of the oxidative metabolites 13-*cis*- and 13-*cis*-4-oxo-retinoic acids were strongly decreased in all patient groups treated with phenytoin, phenobarbital, carbamazepine and ethosuximide, in combination with valproic acid, to levels which were 27% and 6% of corresponding control values, respectively. Little change was observed with all-*trans*-retinoic acid except in one patient group treated with valproic acid-ethosuximide co-therapy where increased levels of this retinoid were found. Our study indicates that therapy with antiepileptic agents can have a profound effect on endogenous retinoid metabolism. Because of the importance of retinoids for signalling crucial biological events during embryonic development, altered retinoid metabolism may be an important factor in antiepileptic drug teratogenesis.

The coadministration of phenobarbital drastically decreased plasma levels of 13-*cis*-retinoic acid and its 4-oxo-metabolite. Phenytoin and carbamazepine may have acted similarly to phenobarbital in the reduction of endogenous retinoids. It is interesting to speculate why the levels of all-*trans*-retinoic acid were not significantly altered in these patients by administration of the inducing antiepileptic agents. It may be that the coadministered valproic acid, previously shown to be an inhibitor of several enzymatic reactions, may have offset the inducing activity of the other anticonvulsants.

ACKNOWLEDGEMENT

The work in our laboratory was supported by grants from the Deutsche Forschungsgemeinschaft (C-6, Sfb 174), from the BgVV, Berlin (ZEBET), and the European Commission (BIOTECH programme).

REFERENCES

Andrews, J.E., Ebron-McCoy, M., Bojic, U., Nau, H. and Kavlock, R.J. (1995). Validation of an *in vitro* teratology system using chiral substances: stereoselective teratogenicity of 4-yn-valproic acid in cultured mouse embryos. *Toxicol Appl Pharmacol* **132**, 310–316.

Carl, G.F. (1986). Effect of chronic valproate treatment on folate-dedendent methyl biosynthesis in the rat. *Neurochem Res* **11**, 671–685.

Czeizel, A.E. and Dudás, I. (1992). Prevention of the first occurrence of neural-tube defects by periconceptional vitamin supplementation. *N Engl J Med* **327**, 1832–1835.

Daly, L.E., Kirke, P.N., Molly, A., Weir, D.G. and Scott, J.M. (1995). Folate levels and neural tube defects. Implications for prevention. *JAMA* **274**, 1698–1702.

Ehlers, K., Stürje, H., Merker, H.-J. and Nau, H. (1991). Valproic acid-induced spina bifida: a mouse model. *Teratology* **45**, 145–154.

Ehlers, K., Elmazar, M.A. and Nau, H. (1996). Methionine reduces the valproic acid-induced spina bifida rate in mice without altering valproic acid kinetics. *J Nutr* **126**, 67–75.

Elmazar, M.M.A. and Nau, H. (1992). Methotrexate increases valproic acid-induced developmental toxicity, in particular neural tube defects in mice. *Teratogenesis Carcinog Mutagen* **12**, 203–210.

Elmazar, M.M.A. and Nau, H. (1993). Trimethoprim potentiates valproic acid-induced neural tube defects (NTDs) in mice. *Reprod Toxicol* **7**, 249–254.

Elmazar, M.M.A., Hauck, R.S. and Nau, H. (1993). Anticonvulsant and neurotoxic activities of twelve analogues of valproic acid. *J Pharm Sci* **82**, 1255-1258.

Hansen, D.K. and Billings, R.E. (1985). Phenytoin teratogenicity and effects on embryonic and maternal folate metabolism. *Teratology* **31**, 363–371.

Hauck, R.S. and Nau, H. (1989a). Asymmetric synthesis and enantioselective teratogenicity of 2-n-propyl-4-pentenoic acid (4-en VPA9), an active metabolite of the anticonvulsant drug, valproic acid. *Toxicol Lett* **49**, 41–48.

Hauck, R.S. and Nau, H. (1989b). Zu den strukturellen Grundlagen der teratogenen Wirkung des Antiepileptikums Valproinsäure (VPA): 2-en-Propyl-4-pentinsäure, das erste Strukturanalogen mit signifikant höherer teratogener Aktivität als VPA. *Naturwissenschaften* **76**, 528–529.

Hauck, R. S., Wegner, C., Blumtritt, P., Fuhrhop, J. H. and Nau, H. (1990). Asymmetric synthesis and teratogenic activity of (R)- and (S)-2-ethylhexanoic acid, a metabolite of the plasticizer di-(2-ethylhexyl)phthalate. *Life Sci* **46**, 513–518.

Hendel, J., Dam, M., Gram, L., Winkel, P. and Jorgensen, H. (1984). The effects of carbamazepine and valproate on folate metabolism in man. *Acta Neurol Scand* **69**, 226–231.

Jäger-Roman, E., Deichl, A., Jakob, S. *et al.* (1986). Fetal growth, major malformations, and minor anomalies in infants born to women receiving valproic acid. *J Pediatr* **108,** 997–1004.

Laurence, K.M., James, N., Miller, M.H., Tennant, G.B. and Campbell, H. (1981). Double-blind randomised controlled trial of folate treatment before conception to prevent recurrence of neural-tube defects. *BMJ* **282**, 1509–1511.

Lindhout, D. and Schmidt, D. (1986). *In-utero* exposure to valproate and neural tube defects. *Lancet* **1**, 1392–1393.

MRC Vitamin Study Research Group (1991). Prevention of neural tube defects: results of the Medical Research Council vitamin study. *Lancet* **338**,131–137.

Nau, H. (1986). Species differences in pharmacokinetics and drug teratogenesis. *Environ Health Perspect* **70**, 113–129.

Nau, H. and Löscher, W. (1986). Pharmacologic evaluation of various metabolites and analogs of valproic acid: teratogenic potencies in mice. *Fundam Appl Toxicol* **6**, 669–676.

Nau, H., Rating, D., Koch, S., Häuser, I. and Helge, H. (1981a). Valproic acid and its metabolites: placental transfer, neonatal pharmacokinetics, transfer via mother's milk and clinical status in neonates of epileptic mothers. *J Pharmacol Exp Ther* **219**, 768–777.

Nau, H., Zierer, R., Spielmann, H., Neubert, D. and Gansau, C. (1981b). A new model for embryotoxicity testing: teratogenicity and pharmacokinetics of valproic acid following constant-rate administration in the mouse using human therapeutic drug and metabolite concentrations. *Life Sci* **29**, 2803–2813.

Nau, H., Hauck, R.S. and Ehlers, K. (1991). Valproic acid-induced neural tube defects in mouse and human: aspects of chirality, alternative drug development, pharmacokinetics and possible mechanisms. *Pharmacol Toxicol* **69**, 310–321.

Nau, H., Tzimas, G., Mondry, M., Plum, C. and Spohr, H.-L. (1995). Antiepileptic drugs alter endogenous retinoid concentrations: a possible mechanism of teratogenesis of anticonvulsant therapy. *Life Sci* **57**, 53–60.

Ogawa, Y., Kaneko, S., Otani, K. and Fukushima, Y. (1991). Serum folic acid levels in epileptic mothers and their relationship to congenital malformations. *Epilepsy Res* **8**, 75–78.

Robert, E. (1988). Valproic acid as a human teratogen. *Congen Anom* **28**, 71–80.

Smithells, R. W. (1984). Can vitamins prevent neural tube defects? *Can Med Assoc J* **131**, 273–276.

Steegers-Theunissen, R.P.M., Boers, G.H.J., Trijbels, F.J.M. and Eskes, T.K.A.B. (1991). Neural tube defects and derangement of homocysteine metabolism. *N Engl J Med* **324**, 199.

Trotz, M., Wegner, C. and Nau, H. (1987). Valproic acid-induced neural tube defects: reduction by folinic acid in the mouse. *Life Sci* **41**, 103–110.

Turner, S., Sucheston, M.E., de Philip, R.M. and Paulson, R.B. (1990). Teratogenic effects on the neuroepithelium of the CD-1 mouse embryo exposed *in utero* to sodium valproate. *Teratology* **41**, 421–442.

van der Put, N., Steegers-Theunissen, R.P.M., Frosst, P. *et al.* (1995). Mutated methylenetetrahydrofolate reductase as a risk factor for spina bifida. *Lancet* **346**, 1070–1071.

Wegner, C. and Nau, H. (1991). Diurnal variation of folate concentrations in mouse embryo and plasma: the protective effects of folinic acid on valproic acid-induced teratogenicity is time dependent. *Reprod Toxicol* **5**, 465–471.

Wegner, C and Nau, H. (1992). Alteration of embryonic folate metabolism by valproic acid during organogenesis: implications for mechanism of teratogenesis. *Neurology* **42** (suppl. 5), 17–24.

Will, M., Barnard, J.A., Said, M. and Ghishan, F.K. (1985). Fetal hydantoin syndrome: inhibition of placental folic acid transport as a potential mechanism for fetal growth retardation in the rat. *Res Commun Chem Pathol Pharmacol* **48**, 91–98.

Epilepsy and Pregnancy
Edited by T. Tomson, L. Gram, M. Sillanpää and S.I. Johannessen
© 1997 Wrightson Biomedical Publishing Ltd

5

Major Malformations Associated with Maternal Use of Antiepileptic Drugs

E. BETTINA SAMRÉN AND DICK LINDHOUT

MGC-Department of Clinical Genetics and Department of Epidemiology and Biostatistics, Erasmus University Rotterdam and University Hospital Rotterdam/Dijkzigt, Rotterdam, The Netherlands

INTRODUCTION

The estimated prevalence of epilepsy lies between four and ten persons per 1000 in the general population (Shorvon, 1990). About 25% of these are women of childbearing age (Delgado-Escueta and Janz, 1992). With the elimination of discriminatory legislation, an increase in public tolerance and understanding, and the availability of antiepileptic medication, more women with epilepsy are marrying and raising families. It has been estimated that, yearly, about 0.3–0.4% of all children are born to mothers with epilepsy (Dansky and Finnell, 1991).

The attitude towards epilepsy patients has long been one of fear and isolation, and treatments have been available only relatively recently (Yerby, 1992). In the eighteenth and nineteenth centuries, most epilepsy patients were institutionalized, and although this gave physicians the opportunity to study large numbers of epilepsy patients, it did not change the negative image of epilepsy. Potassium bromide, the first antiepileptic drug, used by Sir John Laycock, was actually developed to diminish the sexual drive of epilepsy patients and not to treat their seizures. It was not until the beginning of this century that antiepileptic drugs such as phenobarbital (1912) and phenytoin (1938) became available for the treatment of epilepsy, and this progress continued with the introduction of less sedative drugs such as carbamazepine (1961) and valproate (1964). It has long been thought that sufferers from epilepsy should not reproduce, and in many areas of the United States women with epilepsy could compulsorily be sterilized. In many states it was forbidden for people with epilepsy to marry (South Carolina Penal Code, 1976, quoted in Yerby, 1992). Not until our generation have people with epilepsy been granted the same rights and privileges as nonepileptics.

The improvement of medical treatment together with public understanding of the disease, have led to wider opportunities for women with epilepsy to marry and have children. This has also brought an increasing awareness of the potential dangers of drugs and chemicals to the unborn child (Sabin and Oxhorn, 1956), especially once the teratogenic effects of thalidomide became evident in the early 1960s (McBride, 1961). The first formal investigations came from Germany (Janz and Fuchs, 1964) followed shortly thereafter by reports from the UK, describing a pattern of major and minor anomalies involving orofacial, cardiovascular, and skeletal systems in children prenatally exposed to antiepileptic drugs (Meadow, 1968; Meadow, 1970; Speidel and Meadow, 1972).

Besides an increased risk of congenital malformations in the offspring of women with epilepsy, there also seems to be an increased risk of pregnancy complications (Yerby, 1991). There is an increased risk of obstetrical complications, such as vaginal haemorrhage, anaemia, hyperemesis gravidarum, pregnancy-induced hypertension and preeclampsia, and premature labour (Yerby, 1991; Bjerkedal and Bahna, 1973; Nelson and Ellenberg, 1982; Hill and Tennyson, 1982; Yerby et al., 1985a). A higher frequency of labour induction and artificial labour has been reported (Yerby et al., 1985a); however, others have found that the higher rate of artificial labour could not be explained by a higher frequency of medical indications for such procedures (Hiilesmaa et al., 1985).

About 30% of women with epilepsy will have an increase in seizure frequency during pregnancy (Schmidt et al., 1983). There are several hypotheses to explain this increase such as hormonal (increase in serum oestrogens), metabolic (increased sodium and water retention), psychological (increased stress and anxiety), physiological (sleep deprivation), and pharmacokinetic mechanisms. The last, a decrease of plasma drug concentration, is probably the most frequent cause (Dansky et al., 1982a; Schmidt, 1982). Several mechanisms to explain the decline of antiepileptic drug levels have been proposed, such as intestinal malabsorption (Ramsay et al., 1978), decreased plasma protein binding (Perruca and Crema, 1981; Yerby et al., 1985b), reduced concentration of albumin, and increased drug clearance (Philbert and Dam, 1982; Nau et al., 1981; Janz, 1982a; Eadie et al., 1977; Dam et al., 1979). On the other hand, if the albumin concentration and the protein binding decrease, the plasma levels of unbound drug could remain unaltered, which would not necessitate adjustment of the dose if seizure activity does not increase. Also noncompliance could play a role because of concern about the influence of antiepileptic drugs on the child. Because of the high risks associated with convulsions during pregnancy, both for mother and fetus, monthly monitoring of antiepileptic drug levels has been advised (Levy and Yerby, 1985). Status epilepticus has a high maternal and perinatal mortality. Of 29 reported cases (reviewed by Teramo and Hiilesmaa,

1982), nine of the mothers and 14 of the infants died during or shortly after an episode of status epilepticus. Generalized seizures also have other adverse effects on the fetus, such as hypoxia, observed in fetal heart rate (Teramo *et al.*, 1979) and acidosis (Stumpf and Frost, 1978; Orringer *et al.*, 1977). It has been suggested that such seizures cause structural defects when occurring in the first trimester, or mental retardation when occurring in the third trimester of pregnancy (Janz, 1982a). So far, however, no proof for such a causal relation exists, mainly due to lack of a significant proportion of observations of malformations associated with generalized maternal seizures during the malformation-specific period of pregnancy. Whether partial seizures can have an effect on the fetus is still unknown.

The high risk of complications with generalized seizures is also one of the reasons why it is usually not wise or possible to discontinue medication during pregnancy. Even if it were possible to ensure a complete seizure-free pregnancy without antiepileptic medication, many women do not consult their doctor until several weeks after conception. The slow dose reduction which is necessary to safely discontinue antiepileptic drugs will not prevent exposure of the embryo to the drug during organogenesis. Furthermore, the risk of a grand mal seizure is increased during labour. Although the absolute frequency of a grand mal seizure during delivery of 1–2% is small, the probability is about nine times higher than on average during pregnancy (Hiilesmaa, 1992).

Finally, controversy remains as to whether genetic factors associated with epilepsy itself, maternal seizures, or other complications of pregnancy are responsible for the increased rate of adverse pregnancy outcome, or whether this is exclusively due to a direct teratogenic effect of the drug. With most cases of developmental and growth abnormalities though, interaction between or addition of genetic and environmental factors plays a significant role (Gaily *et al.*, 1990; Granström and Gaily, 1992). Some investigators believe that antiepileptic drugs only induce congenital abnormalities in the offspring of epileptic mothers who are genetically predisposed (Janz, 1982b). Others believe that the severity of the seizure disorder determines whether a child is born with an abnormality, and not its drug treatment (Majewski *et al.*, 1981) but this hypothesis has not yet been confirmed or even corroborated by later reports. Most studies clearly have too small a denominator for effective stratification for maternal epilepsy and seizure types, and for family history. The elucidation of genetic factors in epilepsy by molecular genetic methods may help in future to resolve the contribution of genetic and teratogenic factors in adverse pregnancy outcomes.

EPIDEMIOLOGICAL STUDIES

It remains difficult to determine any single cause, but antiepileptic drugs seem to play an important role in the development of major congenital malformations, regardless of confounding factors such as type of epilepsy.

Many epidemiologic studies have been and are still being performed and, so far, most of them have shown a two- to threefold increase in the risk of congenital malformations in the offspring of epileptic mothers using antiepileptic drugs during pregnancy compared with the general population.

Different types of epidemiological studies have been performed over the past few decades investigating the risks of congenital malformations in the offspring of mothers with epilepsy, with or without antiepileptic drug use during pregnancy, and some of them will be discussed here.

Case–control studies

Case–control studies are an efficient way to study rare outcomes, such as congenital malformations, since the selection procedure focuses on the outcome in which one is interested, and not on all pregnancies of which the majority will have a normal outcome (Hennekens and Buring, 1987). Case–control studies also have disadvantages, for example selection bias and the possibility that the data on exposure, which are collected retrospectively, are incomplete and also subject to bias. Most case–control studies, however, have consistently shown a two- to fourfold increase in prevalence of maternal epilepsy among offspring with major congenital malformations as compared with prevalence of maternal epilepsy in the general population (Dansky and Finnel, 1991; Greenberg et al., 1977; Shapiro et al., 1976; Bertollini et al., 1985; Mastroiacovo et al., 1983). Not all studies controlled for type of epilepsy or seizures, making it difficult to separate the teratogenic effect of antiepileptic drugs from a possible predisposition to structural birth defects genetically related to the maternal epilepsy, or from the teratogenic influence of seizures during pregnancy.

In summary, the studies show a four- to elevenfold increase in risk of orofacial clefts (Erickson and Oakley, 1974; Carter et al., 1980; Lakos and Czeizel, 1977; Källén et al., 1989), a four- to sevenfold increase in risk of congenital heart defects for offspring of mothers with epilepsy (Anderson, 1976; Bertollini et al., 1985), and a causal relationship between valproate use and neural tube defects (odds ratio 21:1) (Dansky and Finnel, 1991; Robert and Guibaud, 1982; Anonymous, 1982; Bjerkedal et al., 1982; Robert and Rosa, 1983; Lindhout and Meinardi, 1984). The relationship between maternal valproate use and open neural tube defects was subsequently confirmed by a prospective multicentre cohort study (Lindhout and Schmidt, 1986).

Cohort studies

Cohort studies, retrospective as well as prospective, are an accurate means to study relatively rare exposures, such as epilepsy with or without antiepileptic drug use during pregnancy. Ascertainment of the cohort is based on exposure factors, and occurs before or independent of the outcome, in prospective or retrospective designs respectively (Hennekens and Buring, 1987). The advantage of cohort studies is that they give an estimate of the absolute and relative risks of an exposed versus an unexposed group. Disadvantages of cohort studies are frequently a lack of sufficient sample size with regard to the outcome of interest, i.e. major congenital malformations, and the possibility of confounding by indication. In addition, in retrospective cohort studies there could be the problem of incomplete data, and in prospective cohort studies loss to follow-up might be a problem.

Several retrospective (Speidel and Meadow, 1972; Fedrick, 1973; Koppe *et al.*, 1973; Lowe, 1973; Bjerkedal, 1982; Bertollini *et al.*, 1987) and prospective (Millar and Nevin, 1973; Monson *et al.*, 1973; Knight and Rhind, 1975; Shapiro *et al.*, 1976; Koch *et al.*, 1983; Jones *et al.*, 1989; Lindhout and Schmidt, 1986; Omtzigt, 1992) studies have been performed. Although these cohort studies differ in methodology and populations studied, they all show a variably increased prevalence of major congenital malformations among the offspring of epileptic women as compared with the offspring of nonepileptic controls (Dansky and Finnel, 1991). Some of these cohort studies have focused on the differences in risk of major congenital malformations between women with epilepsy taking antiepileptic drugs during pregnancy and those not taking antiepileptic drugs (Koppe *et al.*, 1973; Nakane *et al.*, 1982); Dansky *et al.*, 1982b; Monson *et al.*, 1973).

The studies show a two- to threefold increased risk of major congenital malformations in the offspring of women with epilepsy using antiepileptic drugs during pregnancy compared with nonepileptic controls, whereas women with epilepsy without antiepileptic drug use during pregnancy seem to have the same risk as the general population. This last risk estimate may not be completely reliable, since the numbers of untreated women with epilepsy in the studies performed so far were very small, and stratification for type and severity of epilepsy was often not possible. It is as yet unclear whether certain types of epilepsy, independent of the treatment, are associated with a higher risk of major malformations than others. Studies with larger numbers of untreated epileptic women are needed to give more insight into this issue.

MALFORMATION PATTERNS ASSOCIATED WITH ANTIEPILEPTIC DRUGS IN MONOTHERAPY

Although the overall relative risk of major congenital malformations in the offspring of women with epilepsy using antiepileptic drugs is increased two- to threefold compared with the general population, the relative risks of specific major malformations associated with specific drugs may be much higher (Karon, 1980), as is demonstrated by the specific association between valproate use and neural tube defect (see above). In fact, the valproate experience, and to a lesser extent that with carbamazepine, has demonstrated that the teratogenic risk of the different medications may conform to the overall two- to threefold increased risk, but may differ with respect to the pattern and spectrum of the defects.

Hydantoins

Hydantoins in monotherapy have been associated with a pattern of malformations, termed the fetal hydantoin syndrome (Hanson and Smith, 1975; Hanson *et al.*, 1976), consisting of prenatal and postnatal growth deficiency, microcephaly and developmental delay, combined with dysmorphic features such as craniofacial abnormalities, especially hypertelorism, and nail and distal phalangeal hypoplasia. In the study by Hanson and Smith (1975) 11% of the children exhibited this pattern of malformation, while none of the nonexposed controls did. Major congenital malformations associated more often than expected with phenytoin are facial clefts and congenital heart defects (Källén *et al.*, 1989; Anderson, 1976; Annegers *et al.*, 1978). Other defects reported to be associated with hydantoins are urogenital malformations (Hirschberger and Kleinberg, 1975), subcutaneous vascular abnormalities (Kousseff, 1982), ocular malformations (Hampton and Krepostman, 1981), and various types of mainly embryonic tumours (Pendergrass and Hanson, 1976; Blattner *et al.*, 1977; Jiminez *et al.*, 1981). These were predominantly case-reports and most of the cases were simultaneously exposed to other antiepileptic drugs during pregnancy. It is therefore uncertain whether hydantoins were (solely) responsible for these abnormalities.

Several studies investigated whether there exists a dose–response relationship for antiepileptic drugs and major or minor malformations. Concerning phenytoin, some have found a positive dose–response relationship (Dansky *et al.*, 1982c; Dansky *et al.*, 1989), and some have found no dose–response relationship (Nakane *et al.*, 1980; Monson *et al.*, 1973; Kaneko *et al.*, 1988; van Dyke *et al.*, 1988). Furthermore, with the same daily dose and intake, there is a large interindividual variation in plasma concentration of antiepileptic drugs, making it very difficult to draw any conclusions from a dose–response relationship when plasma levels are not known and the actual fetal exposure cannot be sufficiently quantified. Conversely, when only plasma levels are known, but dosages are not, no conclusion can be drawn with regard to dose–response relationship, since plasma levels do not depend only on dose, but also on factors such as comedication and pharmacogenetics. Relatively few studies, though, have assessed maternal antiepileptic drug plasma levels (Dansky *et al.*, 1982c; Lindhout *et al.*, 1992a), and the results of the different studies are not consistent.

Barbiturates (phenobarbital and primidone)

Barbiturates in monotherapy have also been associated with congenital heart defects and facial clefts (Källén *et al.*, 1989; Anderson, 1976; Annegers *et al.*, 1978) and a specific pattern of minor anomalies and dysmorphic features such as growth deficiency and craniofacial and/or limb abnormalities (Rating *et al.*, 1982; Seip, 1976). Concerning dose–response relationship and plasma levels of these antiepileptic drugs, again there are studies that found evidence for a positive relationship (Nakane *et al.*, 1980; Dansky *et al.*, 1982c; Dansky *et al.*, 1989), and studies that did not (Kaneko *et al.*, 1988; Lander and Eadie, 1990).

Carbamazepine

Recent studies have shown an association between carbamazepine and congenital malformations in the same order of magnitude as for barbiturates and phenytoin, but the types of malformations are different. The first neonatal findings documented in association with carbamazepine were abnormal growth parameters such as reduced head circumference, weight and length at birth (Bertollini *et al.*, 1987; Hiilesmaa *et al.*, 1981). Several other studies reported major congenital malformations, such as hip dislocation, inguinal hernia, hypospadias, congenital heart defect and neural tube defects (Granström and Hiilesmaa, 1982; Markestad *et al.*, 1984; Lindhout *et al.*, 1992a; Wladimiroff *et al.*, 1988). The first suggestion of a possible association between carbamazepine and neural tube defects came from a study in 1984 (Lindhout and Meinardi). Subsequently, Rosa (1991) observed eight cases of spina bifida among 1307 carbamazepine-monotherapy-exposed pregnancies in a collection of several cohort studies, giving rise to a two- to tenfold increase in risk, as compared with the general population prevalence of neural tube defects which varies in the corresponding general populations from 0.05 to 0.3%. The risk of spina bifida associated with carbamazepine was recently confirmed in a study in which nine out of 3635 children of epileptic mothers were born with spina bifida, and of whom six had used carbamazepine during pregnancy (Källén, 1994). In this Swedish study, most of the infants with spina bifida were identified in the period from 1984 to 1986. The most probable reason why no new cases were identified after this period is the increased use of prenatal diagnosis because of treated maternal epilepsy. Cases of neural tube defects prenatally diagnosed and followed by termination of the pregnancy, if they had occurred, were not ascertained in this study which used data from a registry of deliveries only.

Even though the studies so far suggest that carbamazepine use in pregnancy increases the risk of spina bifida, due to small numbers of affected children the results are not (yet?) statistically significant. The individual risk of spina bifida for infants exposed to carbamazepine during pregnancy is estimated to be 0.5–1.0%, and prenatal diagnosis has therefore been recommended (Gladstone *et al.*, 1992; Hiilesmaa, 1992).

Whether a dose–response relationship for carbamazepine use and congenital malformations exists is still a subject of discussion (Omtzigt *et al.*, 1993). In the study by Lindhout *et al.* (1992a), pregnancies with abnormal outcome were associated with higher serum levels of carbamazepine. However, these abnormal outcomes could also have been associated with an increased seizure frequency, since serum levels were increased only for those women with an increased seizure frequency who delivered a child with a malformation.

Valproate

The initial report of a possible teratogenic effect of valproate was published in 1980 by Dalens *et al*. Shortly afterwards this was followed by several case-reports of infants with congenital malformations, such as craniofacial, skeletal, cardiovascular, urogenital, cerebral and open neural tube defects (Gomez, 1980; Robert and Guibaud, 1982; Stanley and Chambers, 1982). Valproate exposure was later also associated with a combination of facial dysmorphic patterns, distinct from those described with phenytoin exposure (DiLiberti *et al.*, 1984; Jäger-Roman *et al.*, 1986). The reports were followed by cohort studies evaluating major malformations such as hypospadias, umbilical and inguinal hernias, cardiovascular defects, skeletal defects and hip dislocation, indeed showing an increased risk for valproate monotherapy, especially with respect to spina bifida (Robert *et al.*, 1986; Rating *et al.*, 1987; Kaneko *et al.*, 1988). A multicentre prospective cohort study demonstrated the prevalence of neural tube defects to be 2.5% in offspring of epileptic mothers using valproate monotherapy in pregnancy, 0.35% in offspring of mothers with epilepsy using other antiepileptic drugs, and 0% in nonepileptic controls (Lindhout and Schmidt, 1986). A relationship between valproate and radial ray aplasia, rib and vertebral anomalies has also been reported (Jäger-Roman *et al.*, 1986; Lindhout, 1985; Lindhout *et al.*, 1992b; Verloes *et al.*, 1990; Koch *et al.*, 1992; Sharony *et al.*, 1993).

Valproate is probably the only antiepileptic drug for which a dose–response relationship has been observed rather consistently. A higher daily dose or a higher peak dose seem to increase the risk of major congenital malformations, irrespective of seizure frequency during pregnancy (Lindhout *et al.*, 1992a; Rating *et al.*, 1987; Omtzigt *et al.*, 1992a; Omtzigt *et al.*, 1992c).

Ethosuximide

Almost all antiepileptic drugs have been associated with congenital anomalies in children of mothers using these drugs during pregnancy. Regarding ethosuximide, major congenital malformations, such as facial clefts, have been associated with this drug, but mainly in combination therapies such as ethosuximide + phenobarbital and ethosuximide + primidone. Neonatal behaviour complications and minor anomalies, though, have also been associated with ethosuximide monotherapy (Kuhnz *et al.*, 1984). Furthermore, Nau *et al.* (1995) have investigated the role of various antiepileptic drugs, in monotherapy or combination therapy, in the vitamin A-retinoid metabolism. Several of the drugs, including the combination of valproate with ethosuximide, induced changes in the levels of endogenous retinoid metabolism products. The effect of ethosuximide monotherapy, however, was not studied. With respect to the level of all-*trans*-retinoic acid, it was only the combination of valproate and ethosuximide that was associated with an increase, and not the combinations of valproate with other drugs but, again, no data on ethosuximide only were presented (Nau *et al.*, 1995).

Benzodiazepines

Initial reports on associations between orofacial clefts and benzodiazepines (diazepam) (Safra and Oakley, 1975; Aarskog, 1975; Laegreid *et al.*, 1990) were followed later by studies that were not able to confirm such associations (Lakos and Czeizel, 1977; Rosenberg *et al.*, 1983; Czeizel, 1987). Benzodiazepines are often used as add-on therapy. In a study by Laegreid *et al.* (1993), the combination of valproate and benzodiazepam was found to be associated in two cases with neural tube defects in combination with more pronounced dysmorphism, compared with children prenatally exposed to valproate monotherapy. The authors interpreted this as an amplifying action of benzodiazepines on valproate teratogenicity.

DOSE–RESPONSE RELATIONSHIP

The establishment of a dose–response relationship between fetal exposure and fetal outcome is one of the basic criteria of teratogenesis according to the principles set by Wilson (1977). These principles include that a teratogenic effect is determined by (a) the specific structure of the chemical agent, (b) the specific genetically determined sensitivity of the exposed species, (c) the specific sensitive period of embryonic and fetal development, and (d) the existence of a dose–response relationship (Wilson, 1977). There are several possibilities for evaluating dose–response relationships in studies of human pregnancy exposures such as to maternal antiepileptic drugs. An optimal study design would include the evaluation of different exposure parameters such as daily dose as a measure for general exposure; highest dose per administration as a measure for peak exposure and an indirect estimate of peak levels in maternal serum; total and free maternal serum levels of the parent drug as well as of metabolites as an indirect estimate of fetal exposure; and amniotic fluid levels of parent drug and metabolites as a more direct and average estimate of fetal exposure. In the optimal design, these measurements would be made preferably in the sensitive period of embryonic development which, however, varies for the different fetal malformations, and would imply frequent sampling of the required body fluids. Such an optimal design is difficult to achieve in clinical practice, and may explain at least some of the inconsistencies between the results of the various studies that have attempted to evaluate dose–response relationships. Indeed, most studies evaluated only one or two of the measures of exposures, only in a minority of pregnancies, and not always in the relevant period of embryonic development. The study by Omtzigt (1992) is an example of what might be optimally feasible under these conditions. Total daily dose and dose per administration during late embryonic and early fetal development were analysed, together with serum and amniotic fluid levels obtained in almost all women at the most feasible time-points in pregnancy, namely at referral for prenatal diagnosis (8–14 weeks) and at the time-point of amniocentesis or ultrasound examination (16–20 weeks).

TERATOGENIC RISK OF ANTIEPILEPTIC COMBINATION THERAPIES

There are indications that the risks of congenital malformations are higher, or sometimes lower, for antiepileptic combination therapies, depending on the type of combination. Some studies have used a drug score, combining the number as well as the dose of antiepileptic drugs prescribed, and observed a higher frequency of congenital malformations with a higher drug score (Nakane et al., 1980; Kaneko et al., 1988). This last study did not take into account the highest dose per administration of the individual drugs, which may be an important risk factor in the case of valproate use. Another limitation of the drug score method is that it does not take into account the influence of specific interactions between the different drugs within a combination. Specific associations with major malformations were found with the combination of phenobarbital + phenytoin + primidone (Dansky, 1989) and carbamazepine + phenobarbital + valproate +/– phenytoin (Lindhout et al., 1982).

The increased risks associated with these antiepileptic drug combinations could possibly be ascribed to interaction between these drugs, causing an increase of potentially teratogenic intermediates, such as epoxide intermediates (Lindhout *et al.*, 1984). Another possible mechanism of teratogenicity of the combination of carbamazepine + phenobarbital + valproate +/– phenytoin has been ascribed to the induction of hyponatraemia, which has been associated with *in vitro* embryotoxicity of patient sera on rat embryos (Lindhout *et al.*, 1986). So far, there have been no studies of human pregnancies that evaluated the risk of hyponatraemia in carbamazepine- and oxcarbazepine-related malformations. Recently, the potential significance of as yet unidentified carbamazepine metabolites in drug combinations of carbamazepine with other antiepileptic drugs was established by an animal experimental study, in which pregnant rodents were exposed to carbamazepine in combination with a cytochrome P-450 inducer (phenobarbital) or a cytochrome P-450 inhibitor (stiripentol) (Finnel *et al.*, 1995).

The risk of major congenital malformations is not always increased with antiepileptic drug combinations, since the interaction of drugs can also work the other way around. A decrease of the plasma level of a potentially teratogenic parent drug or metabolite can reduce the risks of malformations compared with that associated with a drug in monotherapy. An example might be the somewhat lower risk of neural tube defects associated with the drug combination of valproate + phenobarbital, in which case phenobarbital seems to reduce valproate levels by induction of valproate metabolism (Nau, 1986). Indeed, valproate levels and metabolites in human pregnancies were lower with other antiepileptic drug combinations, but the numbers were too small for meaningful evaluation of pregnancy outcome (Omtzigt *et al.*, 1992c).

PRIMARY PREVENTION

A significant decrease in the occurrence of neural tube defects was demonstrated among pregnant women without a prior increased risk for neural tube defects (no previous affected child, negative family history, no maternal diabetes, no antiepileptic drug use), who were preconceptionally using a multivitamin preparation with a low dose of folic acid (0.8 mg/day), compared with women using a preparation of minerals with vitamin C only (Czeizel and Dudás, 1992). Following this study, health authorities from several countries have recommended that all women of childbearing age should be supplemented with a low-dose folic acid, via a tablet (current dosage in The Netherlands: 0.5 mg/day), by promotion of a folic-acid-rich diet, by food fortification, or a combination of these.

Previously, high-dose folic acid supplementation of 4–5 mg/day was recommended for women of childbearing age with a recurrence risk of neural tube defects (MRC, 1991). Although maternal antiepileptic drug use, especially valproate and carbamazepine, has been associated with an increased risk of neural tube defects, and a decreased folic acid level has been associated with adverse pregnancy outcome, including spontaneous abortion in epileptic women using antiepileptic drugs (Dansky, 1989), it is not yet clear whether it is indicated or safe to prescribe these dosages to epileptic women using antiepileptic drugs. It should be kept in mind that no convincing evidence has been found for involvement of folic-acid-related pathways in teratogenesis induced by antiepileptic drugs. The antiepileptic drugs which induce the most marked decrease in folic acid levels, phenytoin and phenobarbital, are not as strongly associated with neural tube defects as valproate and carbamazepine, which have less influence on folic acid levels. Decisions concerning treating women with epilepsy using antiepileptic drugs during pregnancy should therefore await clear evidence from animal experiments and double-blind randomized placebo-controlled clinical trials. There does not, however, seem to be any reason for withholding low-dose folic acid supplementation. Higher doses may be needed only if such women exhibit symptomatic folic acid deficiency or if other concurrent risk factors for neural tube defects exist.

Recently, panthothenic acid supplementation proved to decrease substantially valproate teratogenicity in mice, especially with respect to the neural tube, and not with respect to skeletal defects induced by valproate (Sato *et al.*, 1995). The authors conducted their study on the basis of the hypothesis that valproate-induced side-effects may be partly mediated through lowering of levels of coenzyme A (Thurston and Hauhart, 1993), which is synthesized from panthothenic acid in a number of metabolic steps. Indeed, valproate interferes with fatty acid metabolism, and it may well be that panthothenic acid and carnitine, when supplemented, have a beneficial effect on some of the side-effects of valproate. In the current phase of knowledge, however, we should await the results of more extensive (animal) experimental studies, and focus on the evaluation of the pantothenic acid content of current food intake and frequently used multivitamin supplement in relation to pregnancy outcome, before (high-dose) panthothenic acid supplementation is clinically tested in the human situation of maternal valproate use.

SECONDARY PREVENTION OR PRENATAL DIAGNOSIS OF MALFORMATIONS

The risk of spina bifida in the offspring of mothers using valproate (1–2%) or carbamazepine (0.5–1.0%) in pregnancy is of the same order of magnitude as the recurrence risk after a previous child with a neural tube defect and when a sib of one of the parents has such a defect, respectively. Therefore, in many countries, amniocentesis is performed in week 16 of pregnancy in order to measure the α-1-fetoprotein (AFP) level in amniotic fluid. This level is increased in most cases of open neural tube defect (Omtzigt *et al.*, 1992a). Whether maternal serum AFP screening is a reliable method for detecting valproate-induced spina bifida is doubtful (Omtzigt *et al.*, 1992b).

Another widely used method of prenatal diagnosis of major malformations is structural ultrasound screening, which preferably should be performed between 18 and 20 weeks of pregnancy (Wladimiroff *et al.*, 1988). Prenatal detection of major malformations may help to improve perinatal care, and facilitate the acceptance of such malformations for parents. It may also provide parents with the option of terminating the pregnancy in the case of very severe lethal or nontreatable malformations. The limitations of prenatal diagnosis, though, should be made known to parents, since not all defects can be diagnosed prenatally. Furthermore, when a malformation is detected, it is not always possible to give a prognosis, whereas other malformations, especially mental deficiency, may not be detected until after birth.

Last, but not least, the mental and physical impact of a late termination of pregnancy after amniocentesis or abdominal ultrasound screening should not be underestimated. Perhaps in the future transvaginal ultrasound screening performed in the first trimester may offer the possibility of earlier pregnancy termination, but emphasis should be placed upon primary rather than secondary prevention.

REFERENCES

Aarskog, D. (1977). Association between maternal intake of diazepam and oral clefts. *Lancet* **2**, 921.

Anderson, R.C. (1976). Cardiac defects in children of mothers receiving anticonvulsant therapy during pregnancy. *J Pediatr* **89**, 318–319.

Annegers, J.F., Hauser, W.A., Elveback, L.R., Anderson, V.E. and Kurland, L.T. (1978). Congenital malformations and seizure disorders in the offspring of parental epilepsy. *Int J Epidemiol* **7**, 241–247.

Anonymous (1982). Valproic acid and spina bifida: a preliminary report-France. *MMWR Morb Mortal Wkly Rep* **31**, 565–566.

Bertollini, R., Mastroiacovo, P. and Segni, G. (1985). Maternal epilepsy and birth defects: a case control study in the Italian multi-centric registry of birth defects (IPIMC). *Eur J Epidemiol* **1**, 67–72.

Bertollini, R., Källén, B., Mastroiacovo, P. and Robert, E. (1987). Anticonvulsant drugs in monotherapy. Effect on the fetus. *Eur J Epidemiol* **3**, 164–171.

Bjerkedal, T. (1982) Outcome of pregnancy in women with epilepsy, Norway 1967 to 1978: congenital malformations. In: Janz, D., Bossi, L., Dam, M., Helge, H., Richens, A. and Schmidt, D. (Eds), *Epilepsy, Pregnancy and the Child*. Raven Press, New York, pp. 289–295.

Bjerkedal, T. and Bahna, S.L. (1973). The course and outcome of pregnancy in women with epilepsy. *Acta Obstet Gynecol Scand* **52**, 245–248.

Bjerkedal, T., Czeizel, A., Goujard, J. *et al.* (1982) Valproic acid and spina bifida. *Lancet* **2**, 1096.

Blattner, W.A., Henson, D.E., Young, R.C. and Fraumeni, J.F. (1977). Malignant mesenchymoma and birth defects. *JAMA* **238**, 334–335.

Carter, P.L., Montague, J.C. and Buffalo, M.D. (1980). Preliminary data relative to the correlation of medications taken during the first trimester of pregnancy and subsequent cleft palate. *Folia Phoniat* **32**, 298–308.

Czeizel, A.E. (1987) Lack of evidence of teratogenicity of benzodiazepine drugs in Hungary. *Reprod Toxicol* **1**, 183–188.

Czeizel, A.E. and Dudás, I. (1992). Prevention of first occurrence of neural tube defects by periconceptional vitamin supplementation. *N Engl J Med* **327**, 1832–1835.

Dalens, B., Raynaud, E.J. and Gaulme, J. (1980). Teratogenicity of valproic acid. *J Pediatr* **97**, 332–333.

Dam, M., Christiansen, J., Munck, O. and Mygind, K.I. (1979). Antiepileptic drugs: metabolism in pregnancy. *Clin Pharmacokinet* **4**, 53–62.

Dansky, L.V. (1989) Outcome of pregnancy in epileptic women: a prospective evaluation of genetic and environmental risk factors. [Thesis]. McGill University, Montreal.

Dansky, L.V. and Finnell, L.V. (1991). Parental epilepsy, anticonvulsant drugs, and reproductive outcome: epidemiological and experimental findings spanning three decades; 2: human studies. *Reprod Toxicol* **5**, 301–335.

Dansky, L.V., Anderman, E., Sherwin, A.L. and Andermann, F. (1982a). Plasma levels of phenytoin during pregnancy and the puerperium. In: Janz, D., Dam, M., Richens, A., Bossi, L., Helge, H. and Schmidt, D. (Eds), *Epilepsy, Pregnancy, and the Child*. Raven Press, New York, pp. 155–162.

Dansky, L.V., Andermann, E. and Andermann, F. (1982b). Major congenital malformations in the offspring of epileptic parents: genetic and environmental factors. In: Janz, D., Dam, M., Richens, A., Bossi, L., Helge, H. and Schmidt, D. (Eds), *Epilepsy, Pregnancy, and the Child*. Raven Press, New York, pp. 223–234.

Dansky, L.V., Andermann, E., Andermann, F., Sherwin, A.L. and Kinch, R.A. (1982c). Maternal epilepsy and congenital malformations: correlation with maternal plasma anticonvulsant levels during pregnancy. In: Janz, D., Dam, M., Richens, A., Bossi, L., Helge, H. and Schmidt, D. (Eds), *Epilepsy, Pregnancy, and the Child*. Raven Press, New York, pp. 251–258.

Dansky, L.V., Wolfson, C., Andermann, E., Andermann, F. and Sherwin, A. (1989). A multivariate analysis of risk factors for major congenital malformations in offspring of epileptic women. *Epilepsia* **30**, 678.

Delgado-Escueta, A.V. and Janz, D. (1992). Pregnancy and teratogenesis in epilepsy. *Neurology* **42** (suppl 5), 7.

DiLiberti, J.H., Farndon, P.A., Dennis, N.R. and Curry, C.J.R. (1984). The fetal valproate syndrome. *Am J Med Genet* **19**, 473–481.

Eadie, M.J., Lander, C.M. and Tyrer, J.H. (1977), Plasma drug level monitoring in pregnancy. *Clin Pharmacokinet* **2**, 427–436.

Erickson, J.D. and Oakley, G.P. (1974). Seizure disorders in mothers of children with orofacial clefts. A case-control study. *J Pediatr* **84**, 244–246.

Fedrick, J. (1973). Epilepsy and pregnancy: a report from the Oxford Record Linkage Study. *BMJ* **2**, 442–448.

Finnel, R.H., Bennet, G.D., Slattery, J.T., Amore, B.M., Bajpal, M. and Levy, R.H. (1995). Effect of treatment with phenobarbital and stiripentol on carbamazepine-induced teratogenicity and reactive metabolite formation. *Teratology* **52**, 324–332.

Gaily, E., Kantola-Sorsa, E. and Granström, M.L. (1990). Specific cognitive dysfunction in children with epileptic mothers. *Dev Med Child Neurol* **32**, 403–414.

Gladstone, D.J., Bologa, M., Maguire, C., Pastuzak, A. and Koren, G. (1992). Course of pregnancy and fetal outcome following maternal exposure to carbamazepine and phenytoin: a prospective study. *Reprod Toxicol* **6**, 257–261.

Gomez, M.R. (1981). Possible teratogenicity of valproic acid. *J Pediatr* **98**, 508–509.

Granström, M.L. and Hiilesmaa, V.K. (1982). Malformations and minor anomalies in children of epileptic mothers: preliminary results of the prospective Helsinki study. In: Janz, D., Dam, M., Richens, A., Bossi, L., Helge, H. and Schmidt, D. (Eds), *Epilepsy, Pregnancy, and the Child*. Raven Press, New York, pp. 251–258.

Granström, M.L. and Gaily, E. (1992). Psychomotor development in children of mothers with epilepsy. *Neurology* **42** (suppl 5), 144–148.

Greenberg, G., Inman, W.H., Weatherall, J.A.C., Adelstein, A.M. and Haskey, J.C. (1977). Maternal drug histories and congenital abnormalities. *BMJ* **2**, 853–856.

Hampton, G.R. and Krepostman, J.I. (1981). Ocular manifestations of the fetal hydantoin syndrome. *Clin Pediatr* **20**, 475–478.

Hanson, J.W. and Smith, D.W. (1975). The fetal hydantoin syndrome. *J Pediatr* **87**, 285–290.

Hanson, J.W., Myrianthopoulos, N.C., Harvey, M.A.S. and Smith, D.W. (1976). Risk to the offspring of women treated with hydantoin anticonvulsants, with emphasis on the fetal hydantoin syndrome. *J Pediatr* **89**, 662–668.

Hennekens, C.H. and Buring, J.E. (1987a). *Epidemiology in Medicine*. Little, Brown, Boston.

Hiilesmaa, V.K. (1992). Pregnancy and birth in women with epilepsy. *Neurology* **42** (suppl 5), 8–11.

Hiilesmaa, V.K., Teramo, K. and Granström, M.L. (1981). Fetal head growth retardation associated with antiepileptic drugs. *Lancet* **2**, 165–167.

Hiilesmaa, V.K., Bardy, A.H. and Teramo, K. (1985). Obstetric outcome in women with epilepsy. *Am J Obstet Gynecol* **152**, 499–504.

Hill, R.M. and Tennyson, L. (1982). Premature delivery, gestational age, complications of delivery, vital data at birth on newborn infants of epileptic mothers: review of the literature. In: Janz, D., Dam, M., Richens, A., Bossi, L., Helge, H. and Schmidt, D. (Eds), *Epilepsy, Pregnancy, and the Child*. Raven Press, New York, pp. 167–173.

Hirschberger, M. and Kleinberg, F. (1975). Maternal phenytoin ingestion and congenital abnormalities: report of a case. *Am J Dis Child* **129**, 984.

Jäger-Roman, E., Deichl, A., Jakob, S. *et al.* (1986). Fetal growth, major malformations, and minor anomalies in infants born to women receiving valproic acid. *J Pediatr* **108**, 997–1004.

Janz, D. (1982a). Antiepileptic drugs and pregnancy: altered utilization patterns and teratogenesis. *Epilepsia* **23** (suppl 1), 53–63.

Janz, D. (1982b). On major malformations and minor anomalies in the offspring of parents with epilepsy: review of the literature. In: Janz, D., Dam, M., Richens, A., Bossi, L., Helge, H. and Schmidt, D. (Eds), *Epilepsy, Pregnancy, and the Child*. Raven Press, New York, pp. 211–222.

Janz, D. and Fuchs, U. (1964). Are anti-epileptic drugs harmful when given during pregnancy? *Germ Med Mon* **9**, 20–22.

Jiminez, J.F., Seibert, R.W., Char, F., Brown, R.E. and Seibert, J.J. (1981). Melanotic neuroectodermal tumour of infancy and fetal hydantoin syndrome. *Am J Pediatr Hematol Oncol* **3**, 9–15.

Jones, K.L., Lacro, R.V., Johnson, K.A. and Adams, J. (1989). Patterns of malformations in the children of women treated with carbamazepine during pregnancy. *N Engl J Med* **320**, 1661–1666.

Källén, B. (1994). Maternal carbamazepine and infant spina bifida. *Reprod Toxicol* **8**, 203–205.

Källén, B., Robert, E., Mastroiacovo, P., Martinez-Frias, M.L., Castilla, E.E. and Cocchi, G. (1989). Anticonvulsant drugs and malformations: is there a drug specificity? *Eur J Epidemiol* **5**, 31–36.

Kaneko, S., Otani, K., Fukushima, Y. *et al.* (1988). Teratogenicity of antiepileptic drugs: analysis of possible risk factors. *Epilepsia* **29**, 459–467.

Karon, J.M. (1980). Interpretation of epidemiologic studies of the relationship among anticonvulsive drugs, epilepsy, and birth defects. In: Hasse, T.M., Johnson, M.C. and Dudley, K.H. (Eds), *Phenytoin-Induced Teratology and Gingival Pathology* Raven Press, New York, pp. 41–57.

Knight, A.H. and Rhind, E.G. (1975). Epilepsy and pregnancy: a study of 153 pregnancies in 59 patients. *Epilepsia* **16**, 99–110.

Koch, S., Göpfert-Geyer, E., Jäger-Roman, E. *et al.* (1983) Antiepileptika währden der Schwangerschaft. Eine prospective Studie über Schwangerschaftsverlauf, Fehlbildungen und kindliche Entwicklung. *Dtsch Med Wochenschr* **108**, 250–257.

Koch, S., Lösche, G., Jäger-Roman, E. *et al.* (1992). Major and minor birth malformations and antiepileptic drugs. *Neurology* **42** (suppl 5), 83–88.

Koppe, J.G., Bosman, W., Oppers, V.M., Spaans, F. and Kloosterman, G.J. (1973). Epilepsie en aangeboren afwijkingen. *Ned Tijdschr Geneeskd* **117**, 220–224.

Kousseff, B.G. (1982). Subcutaneous vascular abnormalities in fetal hydantoin syndrome. *Birth Defects* **18**, 51–54.

Kuhnz, W., Koch, S., Jakob, S., Hartman, A., Helge, H. and Nau, H. (1984). Ethosuximide in epileptic women during pregnancy and lactation period. Placental transfer, serum concentrations in nursed infants and clinical status. *Br J Clin Pharmacol* **18**, 671–677.

Laegreid, L., Olegard, R., Conradi, N., Hagberg, G., Wahlstrom, J. and Abrahamsson, L. (1990). Congenital malformations and maternal consumption of benzodiazepine: a case-control study. *Dev Med Child Neurol* **32**, 432–441.

Laegreid, L., Kyllerman, M., Hedner, T., Hagber, B. and Viggedahl, G. (1993). Benzodiazepine amplification of valproate teratogenic effects in children of mothers with absence epilepsy. *Neuropediatrics* **24**, 88–92.

Lakos, P. and Czeizel, E. (1977). A teratological evaluation of anticonvulsant drugs. *Acta Paediatr Acad Sci Hung* **18**, 145–153.

Lander, C.M. and Eadie, M.J. (1990). Antiepileptic drug intake during pregnancy and malformed offspring. *Epilepsy Res* **7**, 77–82.

Levy, R.H. and Yerby, M.S. (1985). Effect of pregnancy on antiepileptic drug utilization. *Epilepsia* **26** (suppl 1), 25–57.

Lindhout, D. (1985). *Teratogenesis in Maternal Epilepsy: New Aspects of Prevention.* PhD Thesis, Vrije University, Amsterdam, pp. 81–105.

Lindhout, D. and Meinardi, H. (1984). Spina bifida and *in utero* exposure to valproate. *Lancet* **ii**, 396.

Lindhout, D. and Schmidt, D. (1986). *In utero* exposure to valproate and neural tube defects. *Lancet* **i**, 1392–1393.

Lindhout, D., Meinardi, H., Barth, P.G. (1982). Hazards of fetal exposure to drug combinations. In: Janz, D., Dam, M., Richens, A., Bossi, L., Helge, H. and Schmidt, D. (Eds), *Epilepsy, Pregnancy, and the Child*. Raven Press, New York, pp. 275–281.

Lindhout, D., Höppener, R.J.E.A. and Meinardi, H. (1984). Teratogenicity of antiepileptic drug combination with special emphasis on epoxidation (of carbamazepine). *Epilepsia* **25**, 77–83.

Lindhout, D., Meijer, J.W.A., Verhoef, A. and Peters, P.W.J. (1986). Metabolic interactions in clinical and experimental teratogenesis. In: Nau, H. and Scott, W.J. (Eds), *Pharmacokinetics in Teratogenesis, Vol 1. Interspecies Comparison and Maternal/Embryonic-Fetal Drug Transfer.* CRC Press, Boca Raton, Florida, pp. 233–250.

Lindhout, D., Meinardi, H., Meijer, J.W.A. and Nau, J. (1992a). Antiepileptic drugs and teratogenesis in two consecutive cohorts: changes in prescription policy paralleled by change in pattern of malformations. *Neurology* **42** (suppl 5), 94–110.

Lindhout, D., Omtzigt, J.G.E. and Cornel, M.C. (1992b). Spectrum of neural tube defects in 34 prenatally exposed to antiepileptic drugs. *Neurology* **42** (suppl 5), 111–118.

Lowe, C.R. (1973). Congenital malformations among infants born to epileptic women. *Lancet* **i**, 9–10.

Majewski, F., Steger, M., Richter, B., Gill, J. and Rabe, F. (1981). The teratogenicity of hydantoins and barbiturates in humans with considerations on the etiology of the malformations and cerebral disturbances in the children of epileptic parents. *Int J Biol Res Pregnancy* **2**, 37–45.

Markestad, T., Ulstein, M. and Strandjord, R.E. (1984). Outcome of pregnancy in women with epilepsy. *Acta Neurol Scand* **69** (suppl 98), 79–80.

Mastroiacovo, P., Bertollini, R., Morandini, S. and Segni, G. (1983). Maternal epilepsy, valproate exposure, and birth defects. *Lancet* **ii**, 1499.

McBride, W.G. (1961). Thalidomide and congenital abnormalities. *Lancet* **ii**, 1358.

Meadow, S.R. (1968). Anticonvulsant drugs and congenital abnormalities. *Lancet* **ii**, 1296.

Meadow, S.R. (1970). Congenital abnormalities and anticonvulsant drugs. *Proc R Soc Med* **63**, 48–49.

Millar, J.H.D. and Nevin, N.C. (1973). Congenital malformations and anticonvulsant drugs. *Lancet* **i**, 328.

Monson, R.R., Rosenberg, L., Hartz, S.C., Shapiro, S., Heinonen, O.P. and Slone, D. (1973). Diphenylhydantoin and selected congenital malformations. *N Engl J Med* **289**, 1049–1052.

MRC Vitamin Study Research Group (1991). Prevention of neural tube defects: results of the Medical Research Council Vitamin Study. *Lancet* **338**, 131–137.

Nakane, Y. (1982). Factors influencing the risk of malformations among infants of epileptic mothers. In: Janz, D., Dam, M., Richens, A., Bossi, L., Helge, H. and Schmidt, D. (Eds), *Epilepsy, Pregnancy, and the Child.* Raven Press, New York, pp. 259–265.

Nakane, Y., Okuma, T., Takahashi, R. *et al.* (1980). Multi-institutional study on the teratogenicity and fetal toxicity of antiepileptic drugs: report of a collaborative study group in Japan. *Epilepsia* **21**, 663–680.

Nau, H. (1986). Valproic acid teratogenicity in mice after various administration and phenobarbital-pretreatment regimes: the parent drug and not one of the metabolites assayed is implicated as teratogen. *Fundam Appl Toxicol* **6**, 662–668.

Nau, H., Kuhnz, W., Egger, H.J., Rating, D. and Helge, H. (1982). Anticonvulsants during pregnancy and lactation: transplacental, maternal and neonatal pharmacokinetics. *Clin Pharmacokinet* **7**, 508–543.

Nau, H., Tzimas, G., Mondry, M., Plum, C. and Spohr, H.L. (1995). Antiepileptic drugs alter endogenous retinoid concentrations: a possible mechanism of teratogenesis of anticonvulsant therapy. *Life Sci* **57**, 53–60.

Nelson, K.B. and Ellenberg, J.H. (1982). Maternal seizure disorder, outcome of pregnancy and neurologic abnormalities in the children. *Neurology* **32**, 1247–1254.

Omtzigt, J.G.E. (1992). *Epilepsy, Antiepileptic Drugs and Birth Defects.* PhD Thesis, Erasmus University, Rotterdam.

Omtzigt, J.G.E., Los, F.J., Grobbee, D.E. *et al.* (1992a). The risk of spina bifida aperta after first-trimester exposure to valproate in a prenatal cohort. *Neurology* **42** (suppl 5), 119–125.

Omtzigt, J.G.E., Los, F.J., Hagenaars, A.M., Stewart, P.A., Sachs, E.S. and Lindhout, D. (1992b). Prenatal diagnosis of spina bifida aperta after first-trimester valproate exposure. *Prenat Diagn* **12**, 893–897.

Omtzigt, J.G.E., Nau, H., Los, F.J., Pijpers, L. and Lindhout, D. (1992c). The disposition of valproate and its metabolites in the late first trimester and early second trimester of pregnancy in maternal serum, urine, and amniotic fluid: effect of dose, co-medication, and the presence of spina bifida. *Eur J Clin Pharmacol* **43**, 381–388.

Omtzigt, J.G.E., Los, F.J., Meijer, J.W. and Lindhout, D. (1993). The 10,11-epoxide-10,11-diol pathway of carbamazepine in early pregnancy in maternal serum, urine, and amniotic fluid: effect of dose, co-medication, and relation to outcome of pregnancy. *Ther Drug Monit* **15**, 1–10.

Orringer, C.E., Eustace, J.C. and Wunsch, C.D. (1977). Natural history of lactic acidosis after grand mal seizures. *N Engl J Med* **297**, 796–799.

Pendergrass, T.W. and Hanson, J.W. (1976). Fetal hydantoin syndrome and neuroblastoma. *Lancet* **ii**, 150.

Perruca, E. and Crema, A. (1981). Plasma protein binding of drugs in pregnancy. *Clin Pharmacokinet* **7**, 336–352.

Philbert, A. and Dam, M. (1982). The epileptic mother and her child. *Epilepsia* **23**, 85–99.

Ramsay, R.E., Strauss, R., Wilder, B.J. and Wilmore, L.J. (1978). Status epilepticus in pregnancy: effect of phenytoin malabsorbtion on seizure control. *Neurology* **28**, 85–89.

Rating, D., Nau, H., Jäger-Roman, E. *et al.* (1982). Teratogenic and pharmacokinetic studies of primidone during pregnancy and in the offspring of epileptic women. *Acta Pediatr Scand* **71**, 301–311.

Rating, D., Jäger-Roman, E., Koch, S. *et al.* (1987). Major malformations and minor anomalies in the offspring of epileptic parents: the role of antiepileptic drugs. In: Nau, H. and Scott, W.J. (Eds), *Pharmacokinetics in Teratogenesis.* CRC Press, Boca Raton, Florida, pp. 205–224.

Robert, E. and Guibaud, P. (1982). Maternal valproic acid and congenital neural tube defects. *Lancet* **ii**, 937.

Robert, E. and Rosa, F.W. (1983). Valproate and birth defects. *Lancet* **ii**, 1142.

Robert, E., Löfkvist, E., Maugière, F. and Robert, J.M. (1986). Evaluation of drug therapy and teratogenic risk in a Rhône-Alpes district population of pregnant epileptic women. *Eur Neurol* **25**, 436–443.

Rosa, F.W. (1991). Spina bifida in infants of women treated with carbamazepine during pregnancy. *N Engl J Med* **324**, 674–677.

Rosenberg, L., Mitchell, A.A., Parsells, J.L., Pashayan, H., Louik, C. and Shapiro, S. (1983). Lack of relation of oral clefts to diazepam use during pregnancy. *N Engl J Med* **309**, 1282–1285.

Sabin, M.J. and Oxhorn, H. (1956). Epilepsy and pregnancy. *Obstet Gynecol* **7**, 175–179.

Safra, M.J. and Oakley, G.P. (1975). Association between cleft lip with or without cleft palate and prenatal exposure to diazepam. *Lancet* **ii**, 478–480.

Sato, M., Shirota, M. and Nagao, T. (1995). Pantothenic acid decreases valproic acid-induced neural tube defects in mice (I). *Teratology* **52**, 143–148.

Schmidt, D. (1982). The effect of pregnancy on the natural history of epilepsy: review of the literature. In: Janz, D., Dam, M., Richens, A., Bossi, L., Helge, H. and Schmidt, D. (Eds), *Epilepsy, Pregnancy, and the Child*. Raven Press, New York, pp. 3–14.

Schmidt, D., Canger, R., Avanzini, G. *et al.* (1983). Change of seizure frequency in pregnant epileptic women. *J Neurol Neurosurg Psychiatry* **46**, 751–755.

Seip, M. (1976). Growth retardation, dysmorphic facies and minor malformations following massive exposure to phenobarbitone *in utero*. *Acta Pediatr Scand* **65**, 617–621.

Shapiro, S., Slone, D., Hartz, S.C. *et al.* (1976). Anticonvulsants and parental epilepsy in the development of birth defects. *Lancet* **i**, 272–275.

Sharony, R., Garber, A., Viskochil, D. *et al.* (1993). Preaxial ray reduction defects as part of valproic acid embryofetopathy. *Prenat Diagn* **13**, 909–918.

Shorvon, S.D. (1990). Epidemiology, classification, natural history, and genetics of epilepsy. *Lancet* **336**, 93–96.

Speidel, B.D. and Meadow, S.R. (1972). Maternal epilepsy and abnormalities of the fetus and newborn. *Lancet* **ii**, 839–843.

Stanley, O.H. and Chambers, T.L. (1982). Sodium valproate and neural tube defects. *Lancet* **ii**, 1282.

Stumpf, D.A. and Frost, M. (1978). Seizures, anticonvulsants, and pregnancy. *Am J Dis Child* **132**, 746–748.

Teramo, K. and Hiilesmaa, V.K. (1982). Pregnancy and fetal complications in epileptic pregnancies: review of the literature. In: Janz, D., Dam, M., Richens, A., Bossi, L., Helge, H. and Schmidt, D. (Eds), *Epilepsy, Pregnancy, and the Child*. Raven Press, New York, pp. 53–59.

Teramo, K., Hiilesmaa, V.K., Bardy, A. and Saarikoskis, S. (1979). Fetal heart rate during a maternal grand mal epileptic seizure. *J Perinat Med* **7**, 3–6.

Thurston, J.H. and Hauhart, R.E. (1993). Vitamins to prevent neural tube defects. *N Engl J Med* **328**, 1641–1642.

van Dyke, D.C., Hodge, S.E., Helde, F. and Hill, L.R. (1988). Family studies in fetal phenytoin exposure. *J Pediatr* **113**, 301–306.

Verloes, A., Frikiche, A., Gremillet, C. *et al.* (1990). Proximal phocomelia and radial ray aplasia in fetal valproic syndrome. *Eur J Pediatr* **149**, 266–267.

Wilson, J.G. (1977). Current status of teratology. In: Wilson, J.G. and Fraser, F.C. (Eds), *The Handbook of Teratology, Vol 1*. Plenum Press, New York, pp. 47–74.

Wladimiroff, J.W., Stewart, P.A., Reuss, A., van Sway, E., Lindhout, D. and Sachs, E.S. (1988). The role of ultrasound in the early diagnosis of fetal structural defects following maternal anticonvulsant therapy. *Ultrasound Med Biol* **14**, 657–660.

Yerby, M.S. (1991). Pregnancy and epilepsy. *Epilepsia* **32** (suppl 6), 51–59.

Yerby, M.S. (1992). Risk of pregnancy in women with epilepsy. *Epilepsia* **33** (suppl 1), 23–27.

Yerby, M.S., Koepsell, T. and Daling, J. (1985a). Pregnancy complications and outcome in cohort of women with epilepsy. *Epilepsia* **26**, 631–635.

Yerby, M.S., Friel, P.N. and Miller, D.Q. (1985b). Carbamazepine protein binding and disposition in pregnancy. *Ther Drug Monit* **7**, 269–273.

Epilepsy and Pregnancy
Edited by T. Tomson, L. Gram, M. Sillanpää and S.I. Johannessen
© 1997 Wrightson Biomedical Publishing Ltd

6

Minor Anomalies and Effects on Psychomotor Development Associated with Maternal Use of Antiepileptic Drugs

EIJA GAILY

Department of Child Neurology, University of Helsinki, Helsinki, Finland

INTRODUCTION

Maternal epilepsy may affect development of the offspring in several ways. Antiepileptic drugs carry a risk of teratogenicity and seizures during pregnancy may be harmful. Genetic traits associated with epilepsy may contribute to malformations, developmental defects or dysfunction independent of drug exposure. Children of mothers with epilepsy are also at risk for a poorer psychosocial environment than children of parents without epilepsy (Fedrick, 1973).

One possible way of studying teratogenic effects of antiepileptic drugs in human subjects is to look for minor anomalies in the drug-exposed children. Having one minor anomaly is very common (14%) in the general population (Marden *et al.*, 1964). Multiple minor physical anomalies may indicate a more serious underlying defect or a prenatal cause for such a defect and typical anomalies or combinations may suggest specific aetiology (Smith, 1988).

Retrospective studies have described characteristic minor anomalies in children of mothers with epilepsy and connected these anomalies with prenatal exposure to drugs such as phenytoin (Hanson and Smith, 1975), primidone (Rudd and Freedom, 1979) and valproate (DiLiberti *et al.*, 1984). The characteristic minor anomalies include craniofacial and digital features such as epicanthal folds, hypertelorism, short, low-bridged nose, long philtrum and distal digital hypoplasia. These studies are not further discussed here as they allow no estimation of the magnitude of the risk of developmental defects in the offspring of mothers with epilepsy.

PROSPECTIVE STUDIES

In prospective studies on minor physical anomalies and psychomotor development in children of mothers with epilepsy, mothers have been enrolled before or during pregnancy and data on fetal exposure to antiepileptic drugs and seizures have been collected prospectively. A summary of these studies is given in Table 1. Two studies with data from the Collaborative Perinatal Project (Shapiro et al., 1976; Nelson and Ellenberg, 1982) may be considered population-based. The Helsinki study (Granström, 1982; Gaily et al., 1988a,b, 1990; Gaily, 1990) was also population-based while the remaining studies are clinic-based, with data from one or several hospitals. Information on maternal doses and/or serum levels of antiepileptic drugs during pregnancy is available in seven studies (Hanson et al., 1976; Koch et al., 1983, 1992; Kelly, 1984; Gaily et al., 1988a,b; Jones et al., 1989; D'Souza et al., 1991; Yerby et al., 1992). Fujioka et al. (1984) report 'drug scores' that reflect both drug doses and number of drugs taken by the mother during pregnancy. Evaluations of minor anomalies and/or psychomotor development were blinded in the Collaborative Perinatal Project and in the studies by Andermann et al. (1982), Granström (1982), Gaily et al. (1988a,b, 1990), Jones et al. (1989), D'Souza et al. (1991), Yerby et al. (1992) and Steegers-Theunissen et al. (1994). Parents were examined only by Gaily et al. (1988a).

MINOR PHYSICAL ANOMALIES

Eight prospective studies report the number of minor physical anomalies in general or presence of certain characteristic features in children of mothers with epilepsy (Table 1). All studies show an increase of minor anomalies in children of mothers with epilepsy compared with control children or, less distinctly, in drug-exposed children compared with nonexposed children of mothers with epilepsy. Only distal digital hypoplasia (Andermann et al., 1982; Koch et al., 1983, 1992; Kelly, 1984; Gaily et al., 1988a) and possibly hypertelorism (Gaily et al., 1988a) appear to be connected to prenatal exposure to antiepileptic drugs. The association of distal phalangeal hypoplasia with prenatal phenytoin exposure has been confirmed by anthropometric methods (Gaily, 1990; Kelly, 1984). An excess of dysmorphic features, especially epicanthus, was noted not only in the children but also in the mothers with epilepsy (Gaily et al., 1988a).

PSYCHOMOTOR DEVELOPMENT

Eleven prospective studies have reported data on psychomotor development in children of mothers with epilepsy (Table 1). Early (up to age three years) psychomotor development was found to be retarded in children of mothers with epilepsy by six studies while no retardation was observed in three other studies. An association between retardation and antiepileptic drug exposure was found by Koch *et al.* (1983) but not in the larger study by Nelson and Ellenberg (1982). Catch-up development by preschool and school age was noted in two studies.

Results of intelligence testing at age 4–7 years show lower scores in children of mothers with epilepsy. Shapiro *et al.* (1976) and Gaily *et al.* (1988b) found no association with antiepileptic drug exposure while in the study by Fujioka *et al.* (1984) lower intelligence was correlated with higher drug scores and also with partial seizures occurring during pregnancy.

The highest prevalence of mental retardation was found by Nelson and Ellenberg (1982) who included children of mothers with symptomatic seizures caused by systemic illnesses and intoxications. In the other population-based study where only children of mothers with chronic epilepsy were included (Gaily *et al.*, 1988b), the prevalence of mental retardation was very slightly increased with no correlation to drug exposure.

Neuropsychological test results at 5.5 years of age showed that specific cognitive dysfunction with normal general intelligence was significantly more common in children of mothers with epilepsy than in control children (Gaily *et al.*, 1990). There was a significant association with maternal seizures during pregnancy and partial seizure type but no connection with antiepileptic drug exposure.

DISCUSSION

All prospective controlled studies agree that children with epileptic mothers show an excess of characteristic minor anomalies. Epicanthal folds probably have a genetic connection with epilepsy. This is supported by an excess of epicanthus mothers with epilepsy (Gaily *et al.*, 1988a) and earlier observations of epicanthus being more common in patients with epilepsy than in the normal population (Paskind and Brown, 1936). The examination of parents for minor anomalies is obviously necessary for an assessment of the genetic component in the features of the children.

Distal digital hypoplasia is the only minor anomaly that is clearly connected with prenatal exposure to antiepileptic drugs and specifically to phenytoin. Although hypoplasia may occasionally be severe, with total aplasia of nails, most children who have distal phalangeal hypoplasia show very mild clinical signs by radiological criteria.

The risk of cognitive impairment appears to be increased in the offspring of epileptic mothers compared with children with nonepileptic parents. In both prospective controlled studies that reported intelligence scores (Shapiro

Table 1. Prospective studies on minor physical anomalies and psychomotor development in children of mothers with epilepsy.

Authors, year	Subjects		Minor physical anomalies	Psychomotor development < 3 years	Psychomotor development ≥ 3 years	Prevalence of mental retardation	Specific cognitive dysfunction
Hanson et al., 1976	PHT+	104	11% 'FHS'	No data	Tested at 7 years	5.8% in PHT+ 0% in C	No data
	C	100					
Shapiro et al., 1976	AED+	152	No data	DQ lower in E, AED no effect	IQ lower in E-group. AED no effect	No data	No data
	AED–	192					
	C	28 273					
Nelson and Ellenberg, 1982	AED+	215	No data	No data	Tested at 7 years	6.5% in seizure group, 3.4% in C-group	No data
	AED–	195					
	C	43 926					No data
Andermann et al., 1982	AED+	50	DDH increased in AED+	No data	No data	No data	No data
	AED–	22					
Latis et al., 1982	AED+	18	No data	No difference at 12–24 months	No data	No data	No data
	AED–	1					
	C	19					
Granström et al., 1982	AED+	66	No data	No difference at 18–24 months	No data	No data	No data
	C	66					
Koch et al., 1983, 1992	AED+	116	Increased in AED+, DDH in PHT+	Retarded in AED+ (n=70) catch-up	No data	No data	No data
	AED–	25					
	C	141					

Study	Group	n					
Fujioka et al., 1984	AED+	41	No data	Retarded in E-group	Retarded in E, correlated to drug score & partial seizures Catch-up	No data	No data
	AED–	4					
	C	55					
Nomura et al., 1984	AED+	21	No data	Retarded in AED+	No data	No data	No data
	C	21					
Kelly et al., 1984	PHT+	117	DDH increased in PHT+	No data	No data	No data	No data
	PHT–	54					
Hättig et al., 1987	AED+	70	No data	AED+: lower scores	No data	No data	No data
	C	65					
Gaily et al., 1988a,b 1990	AED+	106	Increased in E, DDH in PHT+	No data	Lower IQ in E-group AED no effect	1.4% in E, ($n=148$). 0% in C	Increased in E, correlated with partial seizures
	AED–	15					
	C	105					
Jones et al., 1989	CBZ+	48	Increased in CBZ+	20% retarded ($n=35$)	No data	No data	No data
	C	70					
D'Souza et al., 1991	AED+	53	Increased in AED+, DDH in PHT+	No significant difference	No data	No data	No data
	AED–	8					
	C	62					
Yerby et al., 1992	AED+	64	Increased in AED+	No data	No data	No data	No data
	C	46					
Steegers-Theunissen et al., 1994	AED+	99	Increased in E, AED no effect	No data	No data	No data	No data
	AED–	20					
	C	106					

PHT, phenytoin; C, control; FHS, fetal hydantoin syndrome; AED +/–, children of mothers with epilepsy exposed/nonexposed to antiepileptic drugs; DQ, developmental quotient; E, children of mothers with epilepsy; DDH, distal digital hypoplasia; CBZ, carbamazepine.

et al., 1976; Gaily *et al.*, 1988b) cognitive impairment was independent of maternal antiepileptic drug therapy. Catch-up development after early retardation noted by some investigators suggests that psychosocial factors may contribute to slow development in some children in the first years of life. In the study by Gaily *et al.* (1988b), the intelligence quotient (IQ) difference between the study and the control group disappeared after adjustment for maternal education (Gaily, 1994), suggesting psychosocial and also genetic effects of maternal epilepsy. The excess of cognitive defects in siblings of epileptic patients (Ellenberg *et al.*, 1985), the excess of mental retardation in the mothers (Nelson and Ellenberg, 1982) and the association of cognitive defects with maternal partial seizure type (Fujioka *et al.*, 1984; Gaily *et al.*, 1990) further suggest that cognitive dysfunction may be genetically transmitted in some epileptic patients and their families.

The risk of mental deficiency is probably slightly elevated in children of mothers with epilepsy. Gaily *et al.* (1988b) reported a prevalence of 1.4% in a population-based study which was very close to the prevalence in the general child population in Finland (Rantakallio and von Wendt, 1986). In the study by Nelson and Ellenberg (1982), the prevalence of mental deficiency in the offspring of mothers with seizures was approximately twofold compared with that of the control population. In that study, however, prevalence was increased by the inclusion of children of mothers with symptomatic seizures from causes that could directly affect the fetal brain. If the estimation had been restricted to children of mothers with chronic epilepsy only, the prevalence would probably have been somewhat lower.

Although retrospective studies report that children with characteristic features after prenatal antiepileptic drug exposure often also have mental deficiency (Hanson *et al.*, 1976), none of the minor anomalies found in excess in children of mothers with epilepsy has been associated with cognitive impairment when studied prospectively (Kelly, 1984; Gaily *et al.*, 1988b; Gaily, 1990).

Concluding from prospective controlled data, the risk of serious developmental defects in children with epileptic mothers is only slightly increased. It is important to note, however, that at least in the Helsinki study (Gaily *et al.*, 1988a,b), monotherapy was common and very high drug levels were rare. Polytherapy and/or toxic drug levels of the mother and defective detoxification capacity in the fetus (Lindhout, 1992) result in an accumulation of teratogenic drug metabolites and may significantly increase the risk for serious defects.

REFERENCES

Andermann, E., Dansky, L.V., Andermann, F., Loughnan, P.M. and Gibbons, J. (1982). Minor congenital malformations and dermatoglyphic alterations in the offspring of epileptic women: a clinical investigation of the teratogenic effects of anticonvulsant medication. In: Janz, D., Dam, M., Richens, A., Bossi, L., Helge, H. and Schmidt, D. (Eds). *Epilepsy, Pregnancy, and the Child*. Raven Press, New York, pp. 235–249.

DiLiberti, J.H., Farndon, P.A., Denis, N.R. and Curry, C.J.R. (1984). The fetal valproate syndrome. *Am J Med Genet* **19**, 473–481.

D'Souza, S.W., Robertson, I.G., Donnai, D. and Mawer, G. (1991). Fetal phenytoin exposure, hypoplastic nails, and jitteriness. *Arch Dis Child* **65**, 320–324.

Ellenberg, J.H., Hirtz, D.G. and Nelson, K.B. (1985). Do seizures in the children cause intellectual deterioration? *N Engl J Med* **314**, 1085–1088.

Fedrick, J. (1973). Epilepsy and pregnancy: a report from the Oxford Record Linkage Study. *BMJ* **2**, 442–448.

Fujioka, K., Kaneko, S., Hirano, T. *et al.* (1984). A study of the psychomotor development of the offspring of epileptic mothers. In: Sato, T. and Shinagawa, S. (Eds). *Antiepileptic Drugs and Pregnancy*. Excerpta Medica, Amsterdam, pp. 196–206.

Gaily, E. (1990). Distal phalangeal hypoplasia in children with prenatal phenytoin exposure: results of a controlled anthropometric study. *Am J Med Genet* **35**, 574–578.

Gaily, E. (1994). Effect of maternal epilepsy and antiepileptic drug treatment on cognitive development and minor anomalies in the offspring. In: Seki, T. (Ed.), *Brain Damage Associated With Prenatal Environmental Factors*. Japanese Organizing Committee of the 6th International Symposium on Developmental Disabilities, Sanyo Kogiyo Ltd, Tokyo, pp. 105–112.

Gaily, E., Granström, M.L., Hiilesmaa, V. and Bardy, A. (1988a). Minor anomalies in offspring of epileptic mothers. *J Pediatr* **112**, 520–529.

Gaily, E., Kantola-Sorsa, E. and Granström, M.L. (1988b). Intelligence of children of epileptic mothers. *J Pediatr* **113**, 667–684.

Gaily, E., Kantola-Sorsa, E. and Granström, M.L. (1990). Specific cognitive dysfunction in children with epileptic mothers. *Dev Med Child Neurol* **32**, 403–414.

Granström, M.L. (1982). Development of the children of epileptic mothers: preliminary results from the prospective Helsinki study. In: Janz, D., Dam, M., Richens, A., Bossi, L., Helge, H. and Schmidt, D. (Eds), *Epilepsy, Pregnancy and the Child*. Raven Press, New York, pp. 403–408.

Hanson, J.W. and Smith, D.W. (1975). The fetal hydantoin syndrome. *J Pediatr* **87**, 285–290.

Hanson, J.W., Myrianthopoulos, N.C., Sedgwick Harvey, M.A. and Smith, D.W. (1976). Risks to the offspring of women treated with hydantoin anticonvulsants, with emphasis on the fetal hydantoin syndrome. *J Pediatr* **89**, 662–668.

Hättig, H., Helge, H. and Steinhausen, H.C. (1987). Infants of epileptic mothers: developmental scores at 18 months. In: Wolf, P., Dam, M., Janz, D. and Dreifuss, F. (Eds), *Advances in Epileptology. XVIth Epilepsy International Symposium*. Raven Press, New York, pp. 579–581.

Jones, K.L., Lacro, R.V., Johnson, K.A. and Adams, J. (1989). Pattern of malformations in the children of women treated with carbamazepine during pregnancy. *N Engl J Med* **320**, 1661–1666.

Kelly, T.E. (1984). Teratogenicity of antiepileptic drugs. III: Radiographic hand analysis of children exposed *in utero* to diphenylhydantoin. *Am J Med Genet* **19**, 445–450.

Koch, S., Göpfert-Geyer, I., Jäger-Roman, E. *et al.* (1983). Antiepileptika Während der Schwangerschaft. *Dtsch Med Wochenschr* **108**, 250–257.

Koch, S., Lösche, G., Jäger-Roman, E. *et al.* (1992). Major and minor birth malformations and antiepileptic drugs. *Neurology* **42** (suppl 5), 83–88.

Latis, G.O., Battino, D., Boldi, B. *et al.* (1982). Preliminary data of a neuropediatric follow-up of infants born to epileptic mothers. In: Janz, D., Dam, M., Richens, A., Bossi, L., Helge, H. and Schmidt, D. (Eds), *Epilepsy, Pregnancy and the Child*, Raven Press, New York, pp. 419–423.

Lindhout, D. (1992). Pharmacogenetics and drug interactions. Role in antiepileptic drug-induced teratogenesis. *Neurology* **42** (suppl 5), 43–47.

Marden, P.M., Smith, D.W. and McDonald, M.J. (1964). Congenital malformations in the newborn infant, including minor variants. *J Pediatr* **64**, 357–371.

Nelson, K.B. and Ellenberg, J.H. (1982). Maternal seizure disorder, outcome of pregnancy, and neurobiologic abnormalities in children. *Neurology* **32**, 1247–1254.

Nomura, Y., Takebe, Y., Nomura, Y., Shinagawa, S., Kaneko, S. and Sato, T. (1984). The physical and mental development of infants born to mothers treated with antiepileptic drugs. In: Sato, T. and Shinagawa, S. (Eds), *Antiepileptic Drugs and Pregnancy*. Excerpta Medica, Amsterdam, pp. 187–195.

Paskind, H.A. and Brown, M. (1936). Constitutional differences between deteriorated and nondeteriorated patients with epilepsy. *Arch Neurol Psychiatry* **36**, 1037–1044.

Rantakallio, P. and von Wendt, L. (1986). Mental retardation and subnormality in a birth cohort of 12 000 children in Northern Finland. *Am J Ment Defic* **90**, 380–387.

Rudd, N.L. and Freedom, R.M. (1979). A possible primidone embryopathy. *J Pediatr* **94**, 835–837.

Shapiro, S., Slone, D., Hertz, S.C. *et al.* (1976). Anticonvulsants and parental epilepsy in the development of birth defects. *Lancet* **i**, 272–275.

Smith, D.W. (1988). Minor anomalies as clues to more serious problems and toward recognition of malformation syndromes. In: Jones, K.L. (Ed.), *Smith's Recognizable Patterns of Human Malformation*. W.B. Saunders, Philadelphia, PA, pp. 662–681.

Steegers-Theunissen, R.P., Renier, W.O., Borm, G.F. *et al.* (1994). Factors influencing the risk of abnormal pregnancy outcome in epileptic women: a multicentre prospective study. *Epilepsy Res* **18**, 261–269.

Yerby, M.S., Leavitt, A., Erickson, D.M. *et al.* (1992). Antiepileptics and the development of congenital anomalies. *Neurology* **42** (suppl 5), 132–140.

Epilepsy and Pregnancy
Edited by T. Tomson, L. Gram, M. Sillanpää and S.I. Johannessen
© 1997 Wrightson Biomedical Publishing Ltd

7

Pharmacokinetics of Antiepileptic Drugs in Pregnant Women

SVEIN I. JOHANNESSEN
The National Center for Epilepsy, Sandvika, Norway

INTRODUCTION

An increased risk for seizures during and immediately after labour has been recognized in women with epilepsy, and there is growing interest in the more subtle management of antiepileptic drug (AED) therapy during pregnancy (Schmidt *et al.*, 1982; Yerby, 1987; Delgado-Escueta and Janz, 1992; Crawford, 1993). The reasons for this increased risk for seizures are not fully understood, but many factors including alterations in antiepileptic drug kinetics, weight gain, decreased albumin levels, as well as patient compliance with therapy, have been suspected (Philbert and Dam, 1982a; Levy and Yerby, 1985).

At constant drug dosage the serum level of most AEDs tends to decrease during pregnancy, but returns to prepregnant level within the first month after delivery. This is of clinical importance because low serum levels may provoke seizures.

Longitudinal studies of the pharmacokinetics of AEDs during pregnancy are few since such studies are difficult to perform for technical, ethical and legal reasons. Therefore, limited information is available concerning antiepileptic drug disposition and protein binding during pregnancy (Nau *et al.*, 1982; Perucca and Crema, 1982; Krauer and Krauer, 1983; Leppik, 1988; Sabers and Dam, 1991; Bardy *et al.*, 1990; Johannessen, 1992; Yerby *et al.*, 1992; Tomson *et al.*, 1994a). This is especially the case with regard to the new antiepileptic drugs.

DRUG DISPOSITION

Drug disposition, i.e. absorption, distribution, metabolism and elimination, is the major determinant of the pharmacokinetic profile of any compound. The pharmacological response obtained is, for the majority of drugs, related to the concentration of drug at its receptor sites.

Drug absorption

Gastric tone and motility are reduced during pregnancy resulting in delayed emptying of the stomach. Nausea and vomiting are other symptoms occurring during pregnancy which affect drug ingestion and absorption, especially during the first trimester. Malabsorption has been reported to play a role in single patients with regard to subtherapeutic AED serum levels during pregnancy, but most investigators have not observed this phenomenon (Yerby et al., 1992). A change in AED bioavailability is another possible explanation for subtherapeutic AEDs in pregnancy, but the bioavailability of most AEDs is high. Although bioavailability does decrease slightly during pregnancy, the change does not appear to contribute significantly to the observed decline in AED levels (Dvorchik, 1982).

Drug distribution

There are marked changes in the body composition during pregnancy (Krauer and Krauer, 1983). Factors which could modify drug distribution in pregnancy are the increased plasma volume and the increased cardiac output due to a higher heartbeat frequency and a greater stroke volume. The plasma volume increases by about 50%, and the cardiac output by about 30%. Total body water increases greatly during pregnancy, with intravascular volume and extracellular fluid both showing large increases. The volume of distribution (Vd) rises with increases in extracellular fluid, fat content and the expanding fetal compartment. An increase in total body fluid is responsible for much of the weight gain during pregnancy and has been considered a likely explanation for low AED levels in pregnancy. As plasma volume increases by 50% by the third trimester, the decline in AED levels could be a dilutional effect.

The Vd of a drug relates its plasma concentration to the total amount of drug in the body. A large Vd implies wide distribution and/or extensive tissue uptake. A small Vd indicates a limited distribution with little tissue uptake. The Vd of a drug depends (among other parameters) on the extent of plasma protein binding and body weight and composition.

Drug protein binding

The degree of serum protein binding is an important determinant of drug disposition and response (Notarianni, 1990). The desired therapeutic serum level range for a drug usually refers to total drug concentration, and drug regimens are adjusted to maintain steady-state concentrations based on that total. If the binding of the drug is altered due to a change in plasma composition (altered proteins and/or binding inhibitors), dose adjustments based on the total serum levels may no longer be valid.

The physiological changes that occur in pregnancy include a reduction in the levels of the two major drug binding proteins, albumin and α_1-acid glycoprotein, potentially altering the fraction of free drug. Serum albumin level is decreased during pregnancy, resulting in fewer binding sites for acidic drugs. Therefore, a decrease in drug binding corresponding to the fall in albumin level would be expected. A reduction in serum protein binding capacity correlates positively with gestational age.

The disposition and ultimate biological effect of the drug may be said to be 'controlled' by the extent of plasma protein binding, since this is the factor limiting the amount of drug available to leave the vasculature and gain access to receptors, tissues and the various sites of elimination and metabolism. Any significant alteration in plasma protein binding can lead to an altered drug disposition and unexpected pharmacological responses. A further consequence of a change in protein binding also has implications in the application of therapeutic drug monitoring. Routine drug analysis normally measures total (unbound plus bound) drug, and any alteration in the unbound versus bound drug ratio may have implications in calculation of the dose. In normal circumstances, protein binding of a specific drug in different individuals falls within a narrow range. If this relationship is altered, the use of total serum concentration of drug will no longer be valid for dose calculations and/or adjustments (Johannessen, 1995).

A knowledge of the conditions under which changes in the plasma protein binding occur, and the extent of those changes, is valuable in predicting response and possible dose adjustment. During pregnancy there is a continuous and significant change in plasma proteins where dose adjustment may be required. The principal plasma proteins involved in drug binding are albumin, glycoproteins, and lipoproteins. Free fatty acids gradually increase during pregnancy and may displace drugs from protein binding sites (Yerby et al., 1990).

Valproate (VPA) is extensively (average 90%) bound to serum proteins (Johannessen, 1981). The unbound fraction of valproate in serum increases with increasing concentrations as a result of saturation of binding sites. At total concentrations in the upper part of the assumed therapeutic range the unbound fraction may increase by about 50%. Furthermore, VPA can be partially displaced from protein binding sites by circulating free fatty acids, which gradually increase during pregnancy (Nau et al., 1984b). The serum protein binding of VPA is significantly decreased in pregnant women. Up to a twofold increase in the unbound fraction has been observed (Riva et al., 1984). Therapeutic concentrations of other AEDs do not appear to alter VPA binding to a clinically important extent (Patel and Levy, 1979).

Like VPA, phenytoin (PHT) is also extensively bound to serum proteins, the unbound fraction being about 10%. Carbamazepine (CBZ) is bound to a lesser extent, with an unbound fraction of about 25%. The unbound fraction of phenobarbital (PB) and ethosuximide (ESM) is about 50% and 100%, respectively (Johannessen, 1981). The decrease in protein binding capacity will result in increased plasma clearance, giving decreased total serum levels. Other changes in pregnancy, e.g. increases in renal clearance and metabolic capacity, increased tissue binding, altered receptor sensitivity and an increase in body water, may counteract the effect of altered drug binding (Notarianni, 1990).

Drug metabolism

Pregnancy is accompanied by changes in almost every aspect of metabolism. There are a number of changes that occur in the liver during pregnancy, and these affect drug metabolism. Changes in liver enzymes are also likely during pregnancy, but are not well understood.

The drugs are cleared from the body mainly by metabolism, and during pregnancy clearance is accelerated because of increased hepatic activity, as a result of the induction of the hepatic microsomal drug-metabolizing system (Hunter, 1976). Increased circulating progesterone is known to induce the system, whereas oestrogens are strong inhibitors. Thus, an increased metabolic rate of the drug may partly depend upon a balance between the effects of progesterone and oestrogens. The great interindividual variation of plasma clearance observed may be explained by the varying ratio of the hormones among individuals.

In pregnancy and labour the body becomes a complex physiological unit consisting of the mother, the placenta, and the fetus. The fetoplacental unit increases the Vd of drugs which are administered to the mother and also contributes to drug metabolism. During pregnancy the extracellular fluid and tissue volume also expand and might altogether lead to the decrease in serum drug level that is observed with an unaltered drug dosage (Sabers and Dam, 1991).

There is some suggestion that during pregnancy VPA metabolism may be significantly altered. There is an increased clearance of VPA during the third trimester which may have multiple mechanisms. These may simply include increased metabolism of VPA to its metabolites, but there also may be some increased renal clearance.

Several studies have suggested that total VPA levels fall, but that unbound fractions increase during pregnancy (Philbert and Dam, 1982b; Nau et al., 1984a). Later studies support these findings (Koerner et al., 1989; Bardy et al., 1990). Despite an upward dose adjustment in some patients, total VPA levels declined as pregnancy proceeded, especially later in pregnancy and at delivery, but unbound levels did not. Plasma unbound fractions and clearances increased, but intrinsic clearances, which were adjusted for changes in body weight, remained unchanged. These findings suggest that the actual metabolism of VPA is not altered by pregnancy and that the changes in plasma clearance were due primarily to decreased protein binding. The altered binding is probably due not only to changes in albumin concentrations, but also to the increased free fatty acid levels.

These observations suggest that, in a given patient, unbound VPA levels will not change significantly as pregnancy advances if the total daily dose in body weight (mg/kg) is kept constant. However, a dose reduction after delivery may be necessary to avoid toxicity.

For VPA, two to three times daily dosing is recommended, preferably with a slow-release preparation, because teratogenic effects are believed to result from high peak serum levels (Nau et al., 1991).

ESM and clonazepam (CZP) are both eliminated mainly by metabolism. The protein binding of ESM is negligible, while CZP is about 50% protein-bound (Johannessen, 1981). Changes in protein binding during pregnancy are thus unlikely to be of clinical relevance, whereas alterations of the metabolic capacity may affect the plasma levels of CZP and ESM.

Tomson et al. (1990) measured plasma concentrations of ESM and CZP during 10 pregnancies compared with plasma levels obtained in the prepregnant period. The apparent plasma clearance of CZP was slightly increased during pregnancy. The interindividual variability was more pronounced for ESM, with unchanged, increased, or decreased plasma clearance. The variable course of ESM steady-state plasma levels during pregnancy results in unpredictable pharmacokinetics. This can be controlled only with frequent monitoring of plasma levels during pregnancy.

Lander and Eadie (1991) measured steady-state plasma AED levels during 134 pregnancies and the postnatal period. Phenytoin (PHT) dosage had to be increased in 85% of pregnancies in which the drug was received, CBZ dosage in 70%, and PB dosage in 85%, in an attempt to prevent or correct a fall in plasma concentrations of the respective drugs as pregnancy progressed. The altered disposition of the AEDs usually began in the first 10 weeks of pregnancy, and had returned to baseline value within four weeks of childbirth in two-thirds of the women receiving PHT. The return to the nonpregnant situation appeared to be slower for CBZ and PB.

Yerby et al. (1992) reported on changes in the pattern of protein binding during 51 pregnancies of the AEDs CBZ, PHT, PB, and VPA. The mean concentration of all drugs declined as pregnancy progressed, decreasing to the lowest level at delivery and increasing again during the postpartum period. The decline in total levels was greatest for PHT (56%), followed by PB (55%), CBZ (42%), and VPA (39%). All reductions were statistically significant. A decline in unbound AED levels was noted for CBZ (11%),

PHT (31%) and PB (50%). The reduction, however, was only significant for PB. The unbound concentration of VPA actually increased by 25%, but this increase was not significant. These findings, at least those for PHT, CBZ, and VPA, support the hypothesis that concentrations of unbound AED do not fall significantly during pregnancy.

The period of pregnancy during which the decrement of AED levels was greatest was different for each medication. The decline in both the unbound and total concentrations was sharpest during the first trimester for PHT and PB and during the third trimester for CBZ, and declined steadily throughout pregnancy for VPA. The unbound fraction (proportion of unbound-to-bound drug) of all AEDs increased as pregnancy progressed, with the proportion of unbound drug being greatest, as compared with baseline, at the time of delivery. The increase in unbound fraction parallelled the decrease in serum albumin concentration.

Changes in AED serum levels during pregnancy are a function of variation in drug dose, body weight, and serum protein binding. While these three factors explain a proportion of the variability in serum drug levels, others may also be important. Changes in serum PB were evident even when dose, weight and binding are accounted for, which may reflect increased renal blood flow during pregnancy. Changes in serum PHT may reflect the drug's nonlinear kinetics. Additional factors to be taken into account are interindividual variability in drug clearance and the potential influence of drug interactions.

Tomson *et al.* (1994a, b) reported on the pharmacokinetics of PHT and CBZ and its active metabolite, CBZ-epoxide, in a prospective study of 86 pregnant women with epilepsy during the three trimesters compared with kinetics at least 10 weeks postpartum. The changes in total CBZ concentrations were minor, although CBZ levels in the second and third trimesters were significantly lower than those at baseline. The unbound CBZ levels, however, were unchanged compared with baseline levels. Consequently, the unbound fraction of CBZ was significantly increased during the second and third trimesters. Total and unbound plasma CBZ-epoxide levels did not change significantly during pregnancy.

For most, total PHT levels decreased steadily as pregnancy progressed, being only 39% of the baseline level in the third trimester. Unbound PHT levels decreased far less, and a significant decrease, 18% as compared with baseline levels, was noted only during the last trimester. The unbound fraction of PHT levels was significantly increased in the last two trimesters.

Bernus *et al.* (1995) reported on urinary excretions of CBZ, CBZ-epoxide, CBZ-*trans*-diol, 9-hydroxyacridan and 2- and 3-hydroxy-CBZ at various stages of pregnancy, and in the postnatal period in 10 women with epilepsy, four of whom took other enzyme-inducing AEDs. Mean plasma CBZ apparent clearance was increased in pregnancy, but only by virtue of the increased clearance in women with comedication. There was evidence consistent with impaired conversion of CBZ-epoxide to CBZ-*trans*-diol during all pregnancies studied. Clearances of CBZ to the various excretory products studied indicated an increased urinary excretion of unmetabolized drug in pregnancy, an increased formation of oxidative metabolites of the drug, and an inhibition of the epoxide–diol pathway.

THERAPEUTIC DRUG MONITORING IN PREGNANCY

The rationale for monitoring drugs in pregnancy is, of course, the same as that for any patient group. It depends on a strong correlation between the unbound concentration of drug at the receptor site and the drug response. For many drugs variations in patient response are a result of pharmacokinetic rather than pharmacodynamic differences, and in pregnancy these differences are often amplified (Choonara and Rane, 1990; Knott and Reynolds, 1990).

The unbound fraction of VPA in serum increases with increasing concentrations due to saturable binding (Cramer and Mattson, 1979). Due to the marked fluctuations in serum VPA levels, the unbound fraction also changes during a dosage interval, and the dose–concentration relationship of the drug may be nonlinear at higher concentrations (Levy *et al.*, 1981). Since only the unbound fraction is available to produce biological effects at the receptor sites, serum levels of total (unbound and bound) VPA would not be expected to reflect accurately the concentration of pharmacologically active drug, suggesting that optimal therapeutic monitoring should be based upon the measurement of unbound drug (Levy, 1980). However, so far it seems that unbound VPA serum levels are not more useful than total levels in predicting seizure control (Farrell *et al.*, 1986; Kilpatrick *et al.*, 1987). Consequently, monitoring of unbound levels should be reserved for special indications such as pregnancy (Barre *et al.*, 1988).

As discussed above, several pharmacokinetic parameters of AEDs are altered during pregnancy, delivery and puerperium. Total AED serum levels decrease as pregnancy proceeds, but the changes in unbound, active concentration may be insignificant. Thus, it is not necessary to modify drug doses according to changes in total concentrations, but it is important to ensure patients' compliance (Koerner *et al.*, 1989; Bardy *et al.*, 1990).

In conclusion, recent findings indicate that total AED serum levels may be misleading, and that monitoring of unbound levels may be advantageous during pregnancy. Thus, preferably both total and unbound serum levels should be closely monitored (once a month if possible, less frequently in well controlled patients) to determine the lowest effective dose and to avoid the harm of seizures and drugs to the mother and fetus. Monitoring unbound levels is, however, only relevant for highly protein-bound drugs like PHT and VPA. Due to low concentrations of unbound drug, sensitive and reliable analytical methods and quality control programmes are mandatory. After delivery, the serum levels should be monitored for the first month, since a dose reduction may be necessary to prevent toxicity (Sabers and Dam, 1991; Johannessen et al., 1991).

Data for the new AEDs are lacking and the role for therapeutic monitoring of these drugs needs to be established.

REFERENCES

Bardy, A.H., Hiillesmaa, V.K., Teramo, K. and Neuvonen, P.J. (1990). Protein binding of antiepileptic drugs during pregnancy, labor, and puerperium. *Ther Drug Monit* **12**, 40–46.

Barre, J., Didey, F., Delion, F. and Tillement, J.-P. (1988). Problems in therapeutic monitoring: free drug level monitoring. *Ther Drug Monit* **10**, 133–143.

Bernus, I., Hooper, W.D., Dickinson, R.G. and Eadie, M.J. (1995). Metabolism of carbamazepine and co-administered anticonvulsants during pregnancy. *Epilepsy Res* **21**, 65–75.

Choonara, I.A. and Rane, A. (1990). Therapeutic drug monitoring of anticonvulsants. State of art. *Clin Pharmacokinet* **18**, 318–328.

Cramer, J.A. and Mattson, R.H. (1979). Valproic acid: *in vitro* plasma protein binding and interaction with phenytoin. *Ther Drug Monit* **23**, 307–313.

Crawford, P. (1993). Epilepsy and pregnancy. *Seizure* **2**, 87–90.

Delgado-Escueta, A.V. and Janz, D. (1992). Consensus guidelines: preconception, management, and care of the pregnant woman with epilepsy. *Neurology* **42** (suppl 5), 149–160.

Dvorchik, B.H. (1982). Drug disposition during pregnancy. *Int J Biol Res Pregnancy* **3**, 129–137.

Farrell, K., Abbott, F.S., Orr, J.M., Applegarth, A., Jan, J.E. and Wong, P.K. (1986). Free and total serum valproate concentrations: their relationship to seizure control, liver enzymes and plasma ammonia in children. *Can J Neurol Sci* **13**, 252–255.

Hunter, J. (1976). Enzyme induction and inhibition in human pregnancy. In: Richens, A. and Woodford, F.P. (Eds), *Anticonvulsant Drugs and Enzyme Induction*. Elsevier, Amsterdam, pp. 131–133.

Johannessen, S.I. (1981). Antiepileptic drugs: pharmacokinetic and clinical aspects. *Ther Drug Monit* **3**, 17–37.

Johannessen, S.I. (1992). Pharmacokinetics of valproate in pregnancy: mother-foetus-newborn. *Pharm Weekly (Sci)* **14**, 114–117.

Johannessen, S.I. (1995). General principles. Laboratory monitoring of antiepileptic drugs. In: Levy, R.H., Mattson, R.H. and Meldrum, B.S. (Eds), *Antiepileptic Drugs, 4th edn*. Raven Press, New York, pp. 179–187.

Johannessen, S.I., Loyning, Y. and Munthe-Kaas, A.W. (1991). Medical treatment. General aspects. In: Dam, M. and Gram, L. (Eds), *Comprehensive Epileptology*. Raven Press, New York, pp. 505–524.

Kilpatrick, C.J., Fullinfaw, R.O., Burg, R.W. and Moulds, R.F.W. (1987), Plasma concentrations of unbound valproate and management of epilepsy. *Aust N Z J Med* **17**, 574–577.

Knott, C. and Reynolds, F. (1990). Therapeutic drug monitoring in pregnancy. Rationale and current status. *Clin Pharmacokinet* **19**, 425–433.

Koerner, M., Yerby, M., Friel, P. and McCormick, K. (1989). Valproic acid disposition and protein binding in pregnancy. *Ther Drug Monit* **11**, 228–230.

Krauer, B. and Krauer, F. (1983). Drug kinetics in pregnancy. In: Gibaldi, M. and Prescott, L. (Eds), *Handbook of Clinical Pharmacokinetics*. Adis, Balgowlah, Australia, pp. 1–17.

Lander, C.M. and Eadie, M.J. (1991). Plasma antiepileptic drug concentrations during pregnancy. *Epilepsia* **32**, 257–266.

Leppik, I.E. (1988). Pharmacokinetics of antiepileptic drug during pregnancy. *Semin Neurol* **8**, 240–246.

Levy, R.H. and Yerby, M.S. (1985). Effects of pregnancy on antiepileptic drug utilization. *Epilepsia* **26** (suppl 1), 52–57.

Levy, R.H., Bowdle, T.A., Patel, I.H. and Wilensky, A.J. (1981). Variability in valproate binding and clearance: implications in therapeutic monitoring. *Epilepsia* **22**, 240–241.

Nau, H., Kuhnz, W., Egger, H.-J., Rating, D. and Helge, H. (1982). Anticonvulsants during pregnancy and lactation. Transplacental, maternal and neonatal pharmacokinetics. *Clin Pharmacokinet* **7**, 508–543.

Nau, H., Helge, H. and Luck, W. (1984a). Valproic acid in the perinatal period: decreased maternal serum protein binding results in fetal accumulation and neonatal displacement of the drug and some metabolites. *J Pediatr* **104**, 627–634.

Nau, H., Schmidt-Gollwitzer, M., Kuhnz, W., Koch, S., Helge, H. and Rating, D. (1984b). Antiepileptic disposition, protein binding, and estradiol/progesterone serum concentration ratios during pregnancy. In: Porter, R., Mattson, R., Ward, A. and Dam, M. (Eds), *Advances in Epileptology*. Raven Press, New York, pp. 239–249.

Nau, H., Hauck, R.-S. and Ehlers, K. (1991). Valproic acid induced neural tube defects in mouse and human: aspects of chirality, alternative drug development, pharmacokinetics and possible mechanisms. *Pharmacol Toxicol* **69**, 310–321.

Notarianni, L.J. (1990). Plasma protein binding of drugs in pregnancy and in neonates. *Clin Pharmacokinet* **18**, 20–36.

Patel, I.H. and Levy, R.H. (1979). Valproic acid binding to human serum albumin and determination of free fraction in the presence of anticonvulsants and free fatty acids. *Epilepsia* **20**, 85–90.

Perucca, E. and Crema, A. (1982). Plasma protein binding of drugs in pregnancy. *Clin Pharmacokinet* **7**, 336–352.

Philbert, A. and Dam, M. (1982a). The epileptic mother and her child. *Epilepsia* **23**, 85–99.

Philbert, A. and Dam, M. (1982b). Antiepileptic drug disposition during pregnancy: review of the literature. In: Janz, D., Bossi, L., Dam, M., Helge, H., Richens, A. and Schmidt, D. (Eds), *Epilepsy, Pregnancy, and the Child*. Raven Press, New York, pp. 109–114.

Riva, R., Albani, F., Contin, M. *et al.* (1984). Mechanism of altered drug binding to serum proteins in pregnant women: studies with valproic acid. *Ther Drug Monit* **6**, 25–30.

Sabers, A. and Dam, M. (1991). Pregnancy, delivery, and puerperium. In: Dam, M. and Gram, L. (Eds), *Comprehensive Epileptology*. Raven Press, New York, pp. 299–307.

Schmidt, D., Beck-Mannagetta, G., Janz, D. and Koch, S. (1982). The effect of pregnancy on the course of epilepsy: a prospective study. In: Janz, D., Bossi, L.,

Dam, M., Helge, H., Richens, A. and Schmidt, D. (Eds), *Epilepsy, Pregnancy, and the Child*. Raven Press, New York, pp. 39–49.

Tomson, T., Lindbom, U. and Hasselström, J. (1990). Plasma concentration of ethosuximide and clonazepam during pregnancy. *J Epilepsy* **3**, 91–95.

Tomson, T., Lindbom, U., Ekqvist, B. and Sundqvist, A. (1994a). Disposition of carbamazepine and phenytoin in pregnancy. *Epilepsia* **35**, 131–135.

Tomson, T., Lindbom, U., Ekqvist, B. and Sundqvist, A. (1994b). Epilepsy and pregnancy: a prospective study of seizure control in relation to free and total plasma concentrations of carbamazepine and phenytoin. *Epilepsia* **35**, 122–130.

Yerby, M. (1987). Problems and management of the pregnant woman with epilepsy. *Epilepsia* **28** (suppl 3), 29–37.

Yerby, M.S., Friel, P.N., McCormick, K. *et al.* (1990). Pharmacokinetics of anticonvulsants in pregnancy: alterations in plasma protein binding. *Epilepsy Res* **5**, 223–228.

Yerby, M.S., Friel, P.N. and McCormick, K. (1992). Antiepileptic drug disposition during pregnancy. *Neurology* **42** (suppl. 5), 12–16.

Epilepsy and Pregnancy
Edited by T. Tomson, L. Gram, M. Sillanpää and S.I. Johannessen
© 1997 Wrightson Biomedical Publishing Ltd

8

Fetal and Neonatal Disposition of Antiepileptic Drugs

ANDERS RANE
Department of Clinical Pharmacology, University Hospital, Uppsala, Sweden

INTRODUCTION

Little was known about the fate of drugs and the pharmacological response in the human fetus until the thalidomide disaster in the early 1960s (McBride, 1961). This event triggered the development of today's preclinical screening for teratogenic drug effects required by the drug controlling agencies.

Our knowledge about the pharmacological response of the human fetus to drugs has improved only modestly since then. Relatively more information has accumulated in the field of fetal drug metabolism. With a few exceptions, the fetus will be exposed to the same drugs and xenobiotics as the mother is exposed to, either deliberately (drug treatment, drug abuse, 'social drugs', e.g. coffee, cigarette smoke, etc.) or inadvertently (pollutants from energy sources, pesticides, herbicides, etc.). Thus, there is a potential risk of pharmacological or toxic effects in the fetus, since nearly all drugs will be transferred across the placenta.

The pharmacologic or toxic response to foreign compounds is not always mediated by the compounds themselves. Recent research has revealed a large number of drugs that are converted to active or toxic metabolites. Similarly, many polluting xenobiotics, e.g. polycyclic aromatic hydrocarbons (PAH), are biotransformed to reactive metabolites, which have been much discussed in respect of their role in mutagenesis, carcinogenesis and teratogenesis (Nebert *et al.*, 1983). Therefore, the metabolism of each drug must be clarified for the full understanding of its pharmacological and toxic potentials. Increased knowledge in this area may contribute to better understanding and prevention of teratogenic, pharmacologic or toxic drug effects in the fetus.

APPROACHES TO THE STUDY OF DRUG DISPOSITION AND RESPONSE IN THE HUMAN FETUS

The use of *in vitro* preparations of fetal organs is commonly employed for studies of drug–receptor interactions and specific types of pharmacological response.

In vivo studies are restrained by the lack of appropriate noninvasive investigational methods. The ultrasound technique has enabled us to study anatomical features and movements of the fetus in response to environmental influence. Certain biochemical drug responses and drug-binding receptors can be studied in the fetus by the use of noninvasive techniques for analysis of endogenous compounds with nuclear magnetic resonance (Smith *et al.*, 1984). Other methods, such as positron emission tomography (PET), may permit studies of the kinetics of drugs (Lindberg *et al.*, 1985). However, the resolution of these techniques has to be improved for broader applications in studies of pharmacodynamic response in the fetus.

APPROACHES TO THE STUDY OF HUMAN FETAL DRUG METABOLISM

Early studies in the late 1950s revealed that embryonic and fetal tissues from various laboratory animals were devoid of drug-oxidizing capacity (Jondorf *et al.*, 1958). We demonstrated for the first time the presence of the cytochrome P-450 enzymes in the human fetal liver (Yaffe *et al.*, 1970). Extensive investigations by several research groups including our own have described the functional capacity of this enzyme system in a variety of drug oxidations (Rane, 1991). For obvious reasons, most studies were performed in the mid-gestational period (when abortions are permitted), and little is known about these enzymes in the last trimester.

Embryonic omnipotent cells behave in much the same way as differentiated hepatocytes through their capacity to form toxic or teratogenic metabolites early in development (Filler and Lew, 1981). There is reason to believe that this occurs also in the human blastocyst. Initial work in man focused on studies of drug-oxidizing enzyme activities in subcellular fractions of fetal tissues, in particular the liver (Yaffe *et al.*, 1970; Pelkonen *et al.*, 1973). Whereas such studies show the presence of specific enzyme reactions, they provide little information regarding their quantitative importance *in vivo*. Metabolic assays in subcellular fractions do not permit interactions between alternative metabolic pathways competing for the same substrate to take place. Therefore, the approach to using isolated hepatocytes was soon applied for studies of acetaminophen metabolism (see below).

There are obvious ethical and medico-legal restraints to the study of the effects of environmental factors (e.g. drugs) on fetal metabolism in man. Attempts to compare large groups of abortuses from phenobarbital-treated and untreated (control) women have been partly successful (Pelkonen *et al.*, 1973). This approach is seldom possible, and results are blurred by genetic variation in the population. An alternative and better approach is to study environmental influence in cultured human fetal tissues (Peng *et al.*, 1984a) in the absence or presence of drugs in the culture medium. The drug-metabolizing enzyme activities may be assayed and compared after harvesting the cells. The cultures are identical in all respects, and they contain exactly the same ingredients, except for the drug studied. Such experiments in our laboratory have revealed that several drugs and experimental chemical agents may induce important drug-metabolizing enzymes in human fetal hepatocytes (Peng *et al.*, 1984a; Rane and Peng, 1985).

Importantly, in these experiments the drug concentrations may be chosen to reflect the actual therapeutic blood concentrations achieved in treated patients. Many drugs are administered at unreasonably high doses in teratogenicity tests. On the one hand, high doses and high blood concentrations may give malformations and fetotoxic effects that are irrelevant to the 'therapeutic' situation. On the other hand, too low a dose may be given, partly because drug metabolism in many species is more rapid than in man (see Chapter 4). This demonstrates the importance of an appropriate design of the experiment.

These results have a general interest not only for evaluation of mechanisms for triggering of the metabolic reactions during ontogenesis. They are also of interest in relation to the proposed association between genetic constitution and liability to develop specific drug-induced toxicity and teratogenicity (Nebert *et al.*, 1983). An interesting and unique case with a discordant expression of the fetal hydantoin syndrome in heteropaternal twins has been discussed from this point of view (Spielberg, 1982; Phelan *et al.*, 1982).

METABOLISM OF ANTIEPILEPTIC DRUGS IN THE HUMAN FETUS

The metabolism of drugs includes two major steps: phase I reactions and phase II reactions (Table 1). Whereas the phase I reactions modify the drug molecule to make it more polar by oxidation, reduction, etc., the phase II enzymes catalyse the conjugation of the drug molecule or its metabolite with polar endogenous water-soluble moieties. These include glucuronic acid, acetyl groups, glutathione, sulphate groups, etc. The most important enzymes that catalyse these reactions are uridine diphosphoglucuronosyl transferases (UDPGT), *N*-acetyltransferases (NAT), and glutathione *S*-transferases (GST).

Table 1. Major drug metabolic reactions.

Phase I reactions	*Enzymes*
Oxidations	Cytochrome P-450 enzymes: amino acid homology: more than 40% within families, more than 55% within subfamilies
Reductions	
Hydrations	Hydrolases
Phase II reactions	*Enzymes*
Glucuronidation	UDP glucuronosyl transferases
Acetylation	*N*-Acetyl transferases (NAT)
Glutathione conjugation	Glutathione *S*-transferases (GST): classes: Alpha, Mu, Pi,
Theta, etc.	
Sulphation	Sulphate conjugases

The most important enzymes catalysing the phase I reactions are the cytochromes P-450 (CYP). The human CYP system comprises at least 25 members of haeme proteins that are vital for the termination of the effects of drugs and other xenobiotics (Gonzalez, 1990; Nelson *et al.*, 1993). The CYP system is an enzyme superfamily, divided into several families and subfamilies on the basis of gene homology (Table 2). The substrates of these enzymes include numerous drugs and environmental or dietary chemicals, as well as natural steroids, fatty acids, prostaglandins, etc. The major CYP forms in the human liver belong to the CYP1A, CYP2C/2D/2E, and the CYP3A families, of which the last-mentioned is the most abundant (Gonzalez, 1990).

The human fetus is unique in its capacity to catalyse the oxidation of several drugs by the last part of the first trimester (Yaffe *et al.*, 1970; Pelkonen *et al.*, 1973). These enzymes are lacking in the fetal liver of almost all experimental animals. Human fetal liver microsomes catalyse the oxidation of several drugs and contain each of the components of the microsomal electron transport chain in the CYP enzyme system (Rane and Ackerman, 1972; Rollins *et al.*, 1979; Yaffe *et al.*, 1970).

Studies of antiepileptic drugs (AEDs) in human fetal liver microsomes

We have investigated the oxidation of carbamazepine. Carbamazepine was found to be consistently oxidized to its major carbamazepine 10,11-epoxide in a series of fetal liver specimens (Piafsky and Rane, 1978). There was no clear relation between enzyme activity and gestational age. However, the condition of the fetus in relation to the abortion procedure may vary substantially and blur this type of correlation. Also, the genetic variation is an important determinant of enzyme activity.

Table 2. Human cytochrome P-450 (CYP) enzymes.

CYP enzyme (chrom. loc.)		Total P-450 (%)	Variability fold	Polymorphism	Noninvasive marker	Inducers
1A1	(15)		100	Yes		Smoking
1A2	(15)	12	40	?	Caffeine	Smoking
2A6	(19)	4	30	Yes	Coumarin	
2B6	(19)	<1	50			
2C9	(10)	20 (all 2C)	25	Yes	Hexobarbital Tolbutamide Warfarin	Barbiturates Rifampicin
2C8/10	(10)					
2C17–18	(10)					
2C19	(10)	<1	>100	Yes	S-Mephenytoin	
2D6	(22)	3	>100	Yes	Debrisoquine	
2E1	(10)	4	30–50	Yes?	Chlorzoxazone	Ethanol
3A4	(7)	30	15		Nifedipine Erythromycin	Barbiturates Rifampicin
3A5	(7)	only in 25%	>100	Yes		
3A7	(7)					
4A1	(1)					Clofibrate

Enzyme-inducing properties of AEDs, as studied *in vitro*

As expected from clinical experience and knowledge about interactions between AEDs and other drugs, phenobarbitone and phenytoin were both found to induce different reactions. We studied epoxide hydrolases which are ubiquitous enzymes and present at high levels in the liver and adrenals. They serve an important role in the detoxification of epoxides, some of which are reactive and may bind to macromolecules and cause tissue damage. The mutagenic, teratogenic, as well as carcinogenic effects of certain compounds have been ascribed to their conversion to unstable epoxides (Huberman *et al.*, 1971; Pacifici and Rane, 1982).

There was an increase in the activity of two epoxide hydrolase activities in isolated cultured human fetal hepatocytes when phenobarbitone and phenytoin were added to the culture medium for periods of 1–3 days (Peng *et al.*, 1984a; Rane and Peng, 1985). There was a concentration-dependent increase in the hydration of styrene oxide, as well as benzo(a)pyrene 4,5-oxide to the respective glycols at 0.1–2 mM phenobarbitone (Peng *et al.*, 1984a). Phenytoin had an inducing effect at 0.1 mM (Rane and Peng, 1985). Since 0.1 mM of these drugs is just above their recommended therapeutic concentration range, it is conceivable that induction of fetal liver enzymes may also take place in the treatment of pregnant epileptic women. Our findings of short plasma half-lives of AEDs in newborns of AED-treated epileptic women would support this assumption. Phenytoin disappeared from the blood of such newborns at half-lives of 7–34 hours, which is a range

observed in adults (Rane *et al.*, 1974). In another study, the half-life of carbamazepine ranged between 8 and 28 hours, which is comparable with or even
shorter than that seen in adults (Rane *et al.*, 1975).

PHASE II REACTIONS IN THE HUMAN FETUS AND INFANTS

A multitude of enzymes catalyse the phase II reactions (Table 2). *In vitro*
methods to study phase II reactions with AEDs are currently not available
for all reactions. Yet, it is known that glucuronidation, sulphation, acetylation reactions, etc. are important in the metabolism of AEDs. We used
paracetamol (Rollins *et al.*, 1979), harmol (Steiner *et al.*, 1982) and
clonazepam (Peng *et al.*, 1984b) as probe drugs for studies of phase II
reactions in isolated human fetal hepatocytes or microsomes. Paracetamol
has at least three major metabolic pathways: conjugation with UDP-
glucuronic acid or sulphate, and oxidation by the CYP enzyme system
followed by glutathione conjugation.

Human fetal hepatocytes catalysed the sulphation, oxidation, and
glutathione conjugation reactions, whereas glucuronidation was not
detectable. These results were in agreement with the clinical studies in
newborn and older infants, children and adults, demonstrating the continuous developmental change in the pattern of paracetamol metabolism
(Garrettson *et al.*, 1975; Levy *et al.*, 1975; Miller *et al.*, 1976; Howie *et al.*,
1977). Taken together, the studies unequivocally demonstrate that there is a
gradual transition from sulphate-conjugating reactions early in fetal life to
glucuronidation reactions which gain an increasing importance postnatally.
The important conclusion from this study was that the metabolism pattern
in fetal hepatocytes is consistent with results from clinical studies at different ages. Even though there was no glucuronidation of paracetamol, prenatal activity of UDP-glucuronosyltransferase activity may be catalysed with
other substrates such as morphine (Pacifici *et al.*, 1982).

We have also demonstrated the early human fetal maturation of the
important glutathione *S*-transferases (GSTs) that catalyse the inactivation
of unstable chemical compounds, drugs, and drug metabolites. The most
well-known example is paracetamol which is converted to a toxic metabolite (supposedly *n*-acetyl-imidoquinone) when the normal conjugating
processes are saturated at high doses, such as in intoxicated patients. The
fetal pattern of GSTs is somewhat different from that of the adult (Pacifici
et al., 1981; Pacifici *et al.*, 1987). Nevertheless, they are catalysing the
glutathione conjugation of several compounds. This reaction involves the
detoxification of xenobiotics and the respective metabolites. There are
reasons to believe that the GST enzymes serve an important role in the
metabolism of certain AEDs.

CYTOCHROME P-450s IN THE HUMAN FETUS

Ontogenic development of cytochrome P-450s

The early studies in human fetal liver have recently been followed up using new methods in molecular biology. The polymorphic CYP2D6 isozyme does not seem to be expressed until late gestational age, when it is present in about one-third of investigated specimens (Treluyer *et al.*, 1991). In liver specimens from newborns, Treluyer *et al.* (1991) showed that the detection rate increases with age. Their findings were in good agreement with studies in our research group, showing a differential development of the *O*- and *N*-dealkylating enzyme reaction pathways with codeine and dextromethorphan as substrates (Ladona *et al.*, 1991). The former reaction, which is catalysed by CYP2D6, was not measurable in mid-gestation in contrast to the CYP3A-associated *N*-demethylation of these drugs. We have recently confirmed these results using another CYP2D6 substrate, codeine, which is metabolized in adult liver to norcodeine (CYP3A) and morphine (CYP2D6).

Studies of cytochrome-P-450-specific transcripts

The biochemical mechanisms that trigger the development of some fetal/neonatal isozymes are related to transcription factors. Such factors have been associated with the postnatal development of various CYP isozymes in rodents, which do not express these enzymes prenatally (Lee *et al.*, 1994). It was found that the developmentally programmed, tissue-specific transcription of CYP2E1, CYP2C6, and CYP2D5 in rodents is due to expression of

Table 3. Cytochrome-P-450-specific mRNAs
in human fetal liver.

CYP species	Liver specimens[a]	
	Fetal liver	Adult liver
1A1	0/16	3/6
1A2	0/16	4/6
2A6/2A7	0/13	6/6
2B6/2B7	0/16	6/6
2C8–19	6/16	6/6
2D6	4/13	4/6
2E1	0/12	6/6
2F1	0/6	0/9
3A3/3A4	9/16	6/6
3A7	9/16	5/6
4B1	0/12	0/6

Source: Adapted from Hakkola *et al.*, 1994.
[a]No. positive specimens out of total investigated.

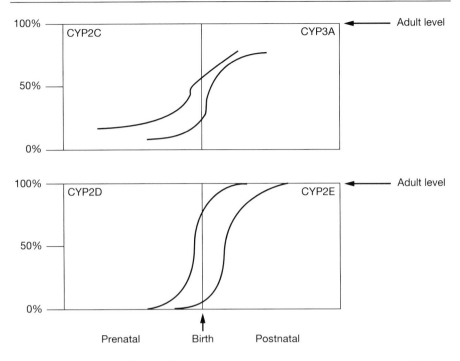

Figure 1. Schematic illustration of perinatal development of cytochromes P-450.

three different transcription factors. With the use of reverse transcriptase polymerase chain reaction methodology for analysis of CYP enzyme-specific mRNAs (messenger ribonucleic acid) we recently demonstrated clear-cut differences in the pattern of CYP gene expression between adult and fetal human livers (Hakkola *et al.*, 1994). As seen in Table 3, certain genes are expressed early in development, e.g. members of subfamilies 3A and 2C. A schematic illustration of the individuality in the development of various CYP species is shown in Figure 1.

Some of the CYP enzymes serve an important role in the metabolism of steroids and other endobiotics. However, future research will have to elucidate the physiological importance of the distinct age-dependent development.

CONCLUSIONS

In the light of the above, it is conceivable that the human fetus is a metabolically very active organism with the potential to detoxify as well as bioactivate a multitude of drugs, including AEDs. The reactions belong to the phase I as well as phase II classes. Thus, the fetus is at risk of being the target of toxic and teratogenic drug effects. Studies in human fetal hepatocytes have demonstrated that drug-metabolizing enzymes may be induced by drugs and other chemical agents. There is reason to believe that a similar induction takes place *in utero* during drug treatment of pregnant women. Two approaches have to be employed for studies of toxic drug effects on the fetus: the experimental *in vitro* approach, as described above, and the epidemiological approach using cohort or case–control data for the statistical assessment of the possible relation between exposure and pregnancy outcome.

ACKNOWLEDGEMENTS

I would like to acknowledge the excellent secretarial and bibliographic help given by Ms Elisabeth Agell. This work was supported by the Swedish Medical Research Council (14X-04496) and the Swedish Cancer Society.

REFERENCES

Filler, R. and Lew, K.J. (1981). Developmental onset of mixed-function oxidase activity in preimplantation mouse embryos. *Proc Natl Acad Sci USA* **78**, 6991–6995.

Garrettson, L.K., Procknal, J.A. and Levy, G. (1975). Fetal acquisition and neonatal elimination of a large amount of salicylate. *Clin Pharmacol Ther* **17**, 98–103.

Gonzalez, F.J. (1990). Molecular genetics of the P-450 superfamily. *Pharmacol Ther* **45**, 1–38.

Hakkola, J., Pasanen, M., Purkunen, R. *et al.* (1994). Expression of xenobiotic metabolizing cytochrome P450 forms in human adult and fetal liver. *Biochem Pharmacol* **48**, 59–64.

Howie, D., Adriaenssens, P.I. and Prescott, L.F. (1977). Paracetamol metabolism following overdosage: application of high performance liquid chromatography. *J Pharm Pharmacol* **29**, 235–237.

Huberman, E., Aspiras, L., Heidelberger, C., Grover, P.L. and Sims, P. (1971). Mutagenicity to mammalian cells of epoxides and other derivatives of polycyclic hydrocarbons. *Proc Natl Acad Sci USA* **68**, 3195–3199.

Jondorf, W.R., Maickel, R.T. and Brodie, B.B. (1958). Inability of newborn mice and guinea pigs to metabolize drugs. *Biochem Pharmacol* **1**, 352–354.

Ladona, M.G., Lindström, B., Thyr, C., Peng, D. and Rane, A. (1991). Differential foetal development of the *O*- and *N*-demethylation of codeine and dextromethorphan in man. *Br J Clin Pharmacol* **32**, 295–302.

Lee, Y.H., Yano, M., Liu, S.Y., Matsunaga, E., Johnson, P.F. and Gonzalez, F.J. (1994). A novel *cis*-acting element controlling the rat CYP2D5 gene and requiring cooperativity between C/EBP beta and an Sp1 factor. *Mol Cell Biol* **14**, 1383–1394.

Levy, G., Khanna, N.N., Soda, D.M., Tsuzuki, O. and Stern, L. (1975). Pharmacokinetics of acetaminophen in the human neonate: formation of acetaminophen glucuronide and sulfate in relation to plasma bilirubin concentration and *d*-glucaric acid excretion. *Pediatrics* **55**, 818–825.

Lindberg, B.S., Hartvig, P., Lilja, A. *et al.* (1985). Positron-emission tomography: a new approach to feto-maternal pharmacokinetics. In: Chiang, C.N. and Lee, C.C. (Eds), *Prenatal Drug Exposure: Kinetics and Dynamics.* NIDA Research Monograph 60, Rockville, MD, pp. 88–97.

McBride, W.G. (1961). Thalidomide and congenital abnormalities. *Lancet* **ii**, 1358.

Miller, R.P., Roberts, R.J. and Fischer, L.J. (1976). Acetaminophen elimination kinetics in neonates, children, and adults. *Clin Pharmacol Ther* **19**, 284–294.

Nebert, D.W., Chen, Y.-T., Negishi, M. and Turkey, R.H. (1983). Cloning genes that encode drug-metabolizing enzymes: developmental pharmacology and teratology. *Prog Clin Biol Res* **135**, 61–79.

Nelson, D.R., Kamataki, T., Waxman, D.J. *et al.* (1993). The P450 superfamily: update on new sequences, gene mapping, accession numbers, early trivial names of enzymes, and nomenclature. *DNA Cell Biol* **12**, 1–51.

Pacifici, G.M. and Rane, A. (1982). Metabolism of styrene oxide in different human fetal tissues. *Drug Metab Dispos* **10**, 302–330.

Pacifici, G.M., Norlin, A. and Rane, A. (1981). Glutathione *S*-transferase in human fetal liver. *Biochem Pharmacol* **30**, 3367–3371.

Pacifici, G.M., Säwe, J., Kager, L. and Rane, A. (1982). Morphine glucuronidation in the human fetal and adult liver. *Eur J Clin Pharmacol* **22**, 553–558.

Pacifici, G.M., Warholm, M., Guthenberg, C., Mannervik, B. and Rane, A. (1987). Detoxification of styrene oxide by human liver glutathione transferase. *Hum Toxicol* **6**, 483–489.

Pelkonen, O., Jouppila, P. and Kärki, N.T. (1973). Attempts to induce drug metabolism in human fetal liver and placenta by the administration of phenobarbital to mothers. *Arch Int Pharmacodyn Ther* **202**, 288–297.

Peng, D., Pacifici, G.M. and Rane, A. (1984a). Human fetal liver cultures: basal activities and inducibility of epoxide hydrolases and aryl hydrocarbon hydroxylase. *Biochem Pharmacol* **33**, 71–77.

Peng, D., Birgersson, C., von Bahr, C. and Rane, A. (1984b). Polymorphic acetylation of 7-amino-clonazepam in human liver cytosol. *Pediatr Pharmacol* **4**, 155–159.

Phelan, M.C., Pellock, J.M. and Nance, W.E. (1982). Discordant expression of fetal hydantoin syndrome in heteropaternal dizygotic twins. *N Engl J Med* **307**, 99–101.

Piafsky, K. and Rane, A. (1978). Formation of carbamazepine epoxide in human fetal liver. *Drug Metab Dispos* **6**, 502–503.

Rane, A. (1991). Variability of drug disposition in infants and children. Concepts and implications. In: Yaffe, S.J. and Aranda, J.V. (Eds), *Pediatric Pharmacology, Therapeutic Principles in Practice.* W.B. Saunders, Philadelphia, PA, pp. 10–21.

Rane, A. and Ackerman, E. (1972). Metabolism of ethylmorphine and aniline in human fetal liver. *Clin Pharmacol Ther* **13**, 652–62.

Rane, A. and Peng, D. (1985). Phenytoin enhances epoxide metabolism in human fetal liver cultures. *Drug Metab Dispos* **13**, 382–385.

Rane, A., Garle, M., Borg, O. and Sjöqvist, F. (1974). Plasma disappearance of transplacentally transferred diphenylhydantoin in the newborn studied by mass fragmentography. *Clin Pharmacol Ther* **15**, 39–45.

Rane, A., Bertilsson, L. and Palmér, L. (1975). Disposition of placentally transferred carbamazepine (Tegretol®) in the newborn. *Eur J Clin Pharmacol* **8**, 283–284.

Rollins, D.E., von Bahr, C., Glaumann, H., Moldéus, P. and Rane, A. (1979). Acetaminophen: potentially toxic metabolite formed by human fetal and adult liver microsomes and isolated fetal liver cells. *Science* **205**, 1414–1416.

Smith, F.W., MacLennan, F., Abramovich, D.R., MacGillivray, I., Hutchison, J.M.S. (1984). NMR imaging in human pregnancy: a preliminary study. *Magn Reson Imaging* **2**, 57–64.

Spielberg, S. (1982). Pharmacogenetics and the fetus. *N Engl J Med* **307**, 115–116.

Steiner, E., von Bahr, C. and Rane, A. (1982). Sulphate and glucuronic acid conjugation of harmol in human fetal and adult liver tissue. *Dev Pharmacol Ther* **5**, 14–20.

Treluyer, J.-M., Jacqz-Aigrain, E., Alvarez, F. and Cresteil, T. (1991). Expression of CYP2D6 in developing human liver. *Eur J Biochem* **202**, 583–588.

Yaffe, S.J., Rane, A., Sjöqvist, F., Boréus, L.-O. and Orrenius, S. (1970). The presence of a monooxygenase system in human fetal liver microsomes. *Life Sci* **9**, 1189–1200.

Epilepsy and Pregnancy
Edited by T. Tomson, L. Gram, M. Sillanpää and S.I. Johannessen
© 1997 Wrightson Biomedical Publishing Ltd

9

Breast-Feeding and Antiepileptic Drugs

ELLEN VINGE

Department of Clinical Pharmacology, Lund University Hospital, Lund, Sweden

INTRODUCTION

Most drugs can pass from the mother's plasma to breast milk, and to some degree back again. The rate and extent of drug transfer into breast milk depend on the maternal plasma levels of the drug, as well as on its physico-chemical properties (for comprehensive review see Anderson, 1991). Drug levels in milk are usually close to those in plasma. However, acidic drugs and drugs with high affinity to plasma proteins tend to have low milk-to-plasma ratios, whereas weakly basic drugs tend to accumulate in breast milk (Atkinson and Begg, 1990). The drug concentration profile in milk essentially follows the plasma concentration curve, but a certain delay can often be seen. Drug concentrations in milk can differ substantially between the first and the last portion of a meal, and between the left and right breast (Matheson and Skjaeraasen, 1988), depending on the fat and protein contents (Fleishaker *et al.*, 1987).

For assessment of the degree of drug transfer to breast milk repeated samples should be taken, preferably from whole portions of milk from both breasts, under steady-state conditions, for estimation of the profile and the area under the concentration–time curve in milk. The milk samples should ideally be matched with plasma samples from the mother, taken during the same time period. Single measurements of milk-to-plasma ratios provide relatively little information.

The total amounts of drugs transferred to the infant via breast milk are usually much smaller than the amounts transferred via the placenta during pregnancy. However, because drug elimination mechanisms are not fully developed in early life, repeated administration of a drug via breast milk, may lead to accumulation in the infant, and pharmacological effects may appear (Nau *et al.*, 1982). Obviously, the degree of accumulation is dependent on the total daily dose in milk. In general, a daily milk intake of 150 ml/kg per day is assumed for calculations. The degree of accumulation is

Table 1. Transfer of antiepileptic drugs via breast milk.

	Milk-to-plasma ratio (range of reported averages)	Estimated dose to the infant (range) (mg/kg/d)	Highest reported plasma level in a breast-fed infant (μmol/l)
Phenytoin	0.1–0.5	0.03–10.70	0.72
Phenobarbital	0.4–0.6	0.60–5.00	36
Primidone	0.7–0.9	0.30–1.90	7
Carbamazepine	0.4–0.6	0.20–0.80	20
Oxcarbazepine	0.5	0.02–0.03	0.4–0.04[a]
Ethosuximide	0.8–1.0	3.00–11.00	280
Valproic acid	0.01–0.1	0.06–1.10	46
Clonazepam	0.3–0.4	0.002	0.015[b]

[a]At age 48–120 h.
[b]Pooled sera from days 2–4.

also dependent on the duration of exposure, the age of the infant, its health status, and any concomitant medication that may cause pharmacokinetic or pharmacodynamic interactions. Since the pharmacokinetics in the infant is extremely important for the net effect of drug transfer via breast milk, studies on milk transfer via breast milk should ideally include drug monitoring of the infant's plasma. However, drug concentration–response relationships may not always be the same in infants as in older children and adults, because of differences in drug distribution and, possibly, because of differences in drug target functions. It should also be borne in mind that all adverse reactions are not concentration-dependent. Type B adverse reactions (i.e. hypersensitivity or idiosyncratic reactions) can occur in sensitive individuals even with very small doses of drugs.

This overview will focus on data based on published pharmacokinetic studies and case-reports. Pharmacokinetic information has been summarized in Table 1. It is obvious that case-reports tend to be biased towards adverse effects, but unfortunately systematic observations in series of breast-feeding epileptic mothers and their infants are essentially lacking, and so are follow-up studies of exposed children. It can be argued that some of the adverse reactions seen in breast-fed infants may be nonspecific, and not related to drug exposure via breast milk. On the other hand, it cannot be excluded that nonspecific symptoms have been unrecognized as adverse drug effects, and therefore were neither reported to the Adverse Drug Reactions Committees, nor described in the medical journals.

PHENYTOIN

Several investigations have shown that phenytoin levels in milk are clearly lower than in the mother's plasma. Reported mean values for milk-to-plasma ratios range between 0.13 and 0.54 (Nau *et al.*, 1982; Bennet *et al.*, 1988, Briggs *et al.*, 1994). Steen *et al.* (1982) calculated from milk concentration data at steady state that the daily dose to the suckling infant would vary between 0.03 and 0.47 mg/kg of bodyweight. Similar figures have been calculated from milk concentration data reported by other groups (see Briggs *et al.*, 1994). The clearance of phenytoin in newborn infants who have been exposed to the drug prenatally is comparable to that in adults (Nau *et al.*, 1982). Excessive accumulation of the drug in infants would therefore not be expected. Reported phenytoin levels in breast-fed infants have been 0.55 μg/ml = 2.2 μmol/l (on the sixth day of life; Rane *et al.*, 1974), 0.46 and 0.72 μmol/l (Steen *et al.*, 1982). In four breast-fed infants investigated by Steen *et al.* (1982) phenytoin was not detectable in plasma. There appear to be no reports on adverse effects associated with phenytoin transferred via breast milk from a woman on phenytoin monotherapy, except for effects in the neonatal period which can be attributed to drug transferred via the placenta. There is one early report on a case of methaemoglobinaemia, drowsiness, and impaired sucking in a 12-day-old girl, which was attributed to phenytoin in the breast milk (Finch and Lorber, 1954). However, the mother also took phenobarbitone (Finch and Lorber, 1954), and methaemoglobinaemia is not a typical adverse effect of either of these drugs.

Conclusion on phenytoin

Relatively small amounts of phenytoin are transferred via breast milk, and serum levels in nursing infants are generally considerably below the therapeutic levels. There appears to be no risk to the nursing infant if phenytoin is given to the mother as monotherapy in conventional doses.

PHENOBARBITAL AND PRIMIDONE

Since primidone is to a large extent metabolized to phenobarbital, these two drugs will be discussed together.

By the 1930s it became clear that barbiturates are transferred to breast milk (Tyson *et al.*, 1938). Milk-to-plasma ratios of phenobarbital have been reported in the range 0.4–0.6 (Nau *et al.*, 1982; Bennet *et al.*, 1988). The average dose of phenobarbital to the infant has been calculated at 0.7–1.6 mg/kg per day, with a range up to 5.0 mg/kg per day (Bennet *et al.*, 1988).

Reported milk-to-plasma ratios of primidone range between 0.48 and 1.15 (Nau *et al.*, 1982; Söderman *et al.*, 1986; Bennet *et al.*, 1988; Meyer *et al.*, 1988). The mean absolute dose of primidone to the infant has been estimated to range from 0.3 to 1.4 mg/kg per day, with a maximum calculated value of 1.9 mg/kg per day (Söderman *et al.*, 1986). The corresponding dose of phenobarbital as a metabolite of primidone has been estimated to be 0.4–1.7 mg/kg per day, with a maximum calculated value of 2.4 mg/kg per day (Söderman *et al.*, 1986).

The elimination of phenobarbital and primidone in neonates varies greatly. Enzyme induction probably plays an important role. Infants who had been exposed to phenobarbital prenatally had generally much shorter half-lives than previously unexposed neonates (100–200 versus 100–500 hours; Nau *et al.*, 1982). Similarly, neonates who had been exposed to phenytoin had shorter half-lives of primidone (around 10 versus 20 hours), whereas maternal use of valproic acid had no such effect (Nau *et al.*, 1982). At four weeks, half-lives of phenobarbital appear to be in the same range as in adults (30–100 hours; Nau *et al.*, 1982).

Due to the slow elimination of phenobarbital, particularly in the first weeks of life, accumulation of the drug to relatively high levels in the infant's plasma is possible. In a 13-day-old infant who suddenly died the post mortem blood concentration of phenobarbital was 8.3 mg/l = 35.7 µmol/l (Juul, 1969). The mother also took primidone and phenytoin, but neither of these drugs could be detected in the infant's blood. In an eight-week-old the serum concentration of phenobarbital was 14.8 µmol/l (Knott *et al.*, 1987). This infant had symptoms interpreted as withdrawal effects when the mother suddenly stopped breast-feeding after seven months, but it should be observed that the mother was also taking other anticonvulsant drugs. In two breast-fed infants, whose mother was treated with primidone 500 mg b.i.d. through both pregnancies, the mean plasma levels of primidone were 4.8 and 7.0 µmol/l, respectively, and the corresponding levels of phenobarbital were 15.3 and 28.9 µmol/l (Söderman *et al.*, 1986). No adverse effects were observed in these infants, but in order to avoid undesired effects the milk was gradually substituted with formula.

Sedation in nursing infants associated with maternal use of phenobarbital was first reported in the 1930s. Tyson *et al.* (1938) noted sedation in two of 21 investigated infants whose mothers had been taking phenobarbital or phenobarbital sodium 1.5 grains (= 100 mg) at bedtime for two to five days, but no effects in 20 infants of mothers who took two grains (= 130 mg) per day. In a later series of 42 infants of 32 mothers, poor weight gain, vomiting and inadequate suckling were reported in some of the infants (Bennet *et al.*, 1988). The mothers were taking phenobarbital and other antiepileptic drugs. It is not clear if plasma levels were measured in the infants.

Conclusion on phenobarbital and primidone

Phenobarbital, given directly or formed from primidone, can accumulate in the nursing infant's plasma. Sedation of nursing infants has been reported. Close clinical monitoring of the infant, supported by monitoring of serum levels, is recommended.

CARBAMAZEPINE

Several groups have reported mean milk-to-plasma ratios of carbamazepine of 0.24–0.6 (Bennet et al., 1988; Briggs et al., 1994), with maximum observed milk concentrations of 4.4 mg/l = 18.6 µmol/l (Meyer et al., 1988). The calculated amounts transferred via breast milk are 0.24–0.38 mg/kg per day (means), maximum 0.83 mg/kg per day (Bennet et al., 1988). Half-lives of carbamazepine in neonates born to mothers who had been treated with carbamazepine as monotherapy during pregnancy were 28 ± 11 hours (Kuhnz et al., 1983), but shorter half-lives were found in infants who also had been exposed to phenytoin before birth (Bertilsson and Tomson, 1986). The apparent volume of distribution of carbamazepine in the neonate appears to be slightly larger than in the adult (Nau et al., 1982). Carbamazepine-epoxide was found at similar concentrations in milk and maternal plasma (Pynnönen et al., 1977), but others found lower levels in milk than in plasma (Kuhnz et al., 1983).

Serum levels of carbamazepine in nursing infants have been found to be around 0.4 mg/ml = 1.7 µmol/l (Briggs et al., 1994), or 1.0 mg/l = 4.2 µmol/l (Kuhnz et al., 1983), but levels up to 4.7 mg/l = 20 µmol/l have been reported (Kuhnz et al., 1983).

Exposure to carbamazepine in utero and via breast milk has been associated with hepatic dysfunction. Cholestatic hepatitis was found in a three-week-old boy whose mother had been on monotherapy with carbamazepine for many years and throughout pregnancy (Frey et al., 1990). The infant's liver function tests normalized after cessation of breast-feeding. Histological functions in a liver biopsy were compatible with a drug-induced hepatitis. The report provides no information on carbamazepine levels in plasma. The authors interpreted the reaction as idiosyncratic hepatotoxicity, which usually occurs within the first six to eight months of treatment, but may occur at any time during exposure to carbamazepine (Stricker, 1992).

Another infant presented with direct hyperbilirubinaemia and high concentrations of gamma-glutamyltransferase (GGT) on the first day of life, which was interpreted as signs of hepatic microsomal enzyme induction in utero (Merlob et al., 1992). The hyperbilirubinaemia resolved in 14 days, but the GGT levels remained above the normal reference for two months. The infant was exclusively breast-fed during nine days, and after that supplementation with formula was introduced in order to reduce drug exposure. The mother continued her medication. The carbamazepine concentration in the infant's serum at age two days was 1.8 µg/ml = 7.6 µmol/l, and at 63 days 1.1 µg/ml = 4.6 µmol/l. The authors suggest that the liver dysfunction was a dose-dependent adverse effect of carbamazepine. However, it is difficult to assess to what extent drug transferred via breast milk contributed to the reaction.

Conclusion on carbamazepine

Breast-feeding is generally considered to be safe when the mother is on carbamazepine monotherapy at normal doses. Carbamazepine concentrations in nursing infants are usually low, and below the level where pharmacological effects should be expected, but may in rare cases induce adverse reactions.

OXCARBAZEPINE

The milk/plasma concentration ratios for oxcarbazepine and 10-OH-carbazepine have been reported to be about 0.5 (Bülau et al., 1988). In a newborn infant who had been exposed to oxcarbazepine during pregnancy, the plasma level of both compounds at delivery were approximately the same as in the mother, i.e. about 0.4 µg/ml for oxcarbazepine and 5.7 µg/ml for 10-OH-carbazepine. The infant was breast-fed from the third day on. At 120 hours after birth, oxcarbazepine levels had declined to about 0.01 µg/ml ($\simeq$ 0.04 µmol/l) for oxcarbazepine and 0.3 µg/ml ($\simeq$ 1.2 µmol/l) for 10-OH-carbazepine (figures estimated from Table 1; Bülau et al., 1988). No data on plasma levels after the neonatal period are available, but it was noted that examination of the child at the age of 13 months showed normal development (Bülau et al., 1988).

Conclusion on oxcarbazepine

The sparse data indicate that neither oxcarbazepine nor its metabolite are likely to accumulate in the infant's plasma.

ETHOSUXIMIDE

Ethosuximide levels in breast milk are similar to those in maternal plasma (Bennet et al., 1988). This is true for both enantiomers of ethosuximide (Tomson and Villén, 1994). As a consequence, relatively high doses of ethosuximide will be transferred via breast milk. It has been estimated that the infant would ingest doses corresponding to 60–100% of the weight-adjusted maternal daily dose (Bennet et al., 1988).

Plasma levels of ethosuximide in one infant exposed to the drug via breast milk over several months rose from 155 µmol/l three days after birth, to 209 µmol/l one month later, and then decreased slowly to about 60 µmol/l after 4.5 months (Rane and Tunell, 1981). In five other infants, individual mean steady-state concentrations in serum ranged from 15 to 40 µg/ml (= 106–283 µmol/l). Corresponding serum concentrations in the mothers were 28–84 µg/ml (= 198–595 µmol/l; Kuhnz et al., 1984). In four of 13 studied infants, sedation was observed in the neonatal period, and five showed hyperexcitability for two to eight weeks. However, all except two of the observed infants were also exposed to other antiepileptic drugs. In one infant, who was fully breast fed for the first four weeks, sedation was observed for five weeks and a lack of weight gain for four weeks. Besides ethosuximide, he was exposed to primidone and valproate. On the other hand, another infant who was prenatally exposed to ethosuximide and primidone and was not breast-fed at all, showed signs of sedation for five days and hyperexcitability for eight weeks (Kuhnz et al., 1984). Others reported that plasma concentrations in three breast-fed infants exposed to ethosuximide were 24–75% of the average maternal concentrations (Söderman and Rane, 1986). These infants had no signs of drug effects (Söderman and Rane, 1986).

Conclusion on ethosuximide

Ethosuximide can be transferred via breast milk to the child in relatively high daily doses, and plasma concentrations in nursing infants can be close to the recommended therapeutic levels. To date, however, there seem to be no data supporting the hypothesis that such high levels would be associated with any substantial risk to the nursing child, but experience is limited. Close monitoring of the child is recommended, and plasma concentration measurements may be helpful.

VALPROIC ACID

Milk concentrations of valproic acid are low, usually less than 10% of the concentrations in maternal plasma (Nau et al., 1982; Briggs et al., 1994). In a study by Nau et al. (1981) the 3-keto-metabolite was also consistently found in human milk at concentrations corresponding to approximately 7% of the maternal serum concentrations, but other metabolites were only found in very low concentrations or were not detected in milk. The absolute dose of valproic acid to the infant has been estimated to be between 0.05 mg/kg per day and 1.08 mg/kg per day, or at maximum 4.7% of the average weight-adjusted maternal dose (Bennet et al., 1988).

Serum valproate levels in one nursing infant during one whole day at three months after delivery were 7.6% of the serum level in the mother (absolute values were not presented; Philbert et al., 1985). There were no adverse effects of valproate in this infant, nor in three other infants exposed to valproate via breast milk during the first three months from birth (Philbert et al., 1985). In a three-month-old suckling, whose mother was treated with sodium valproate 600 mg b.i.d., the serum concentration of valproic acid was 46 µmol/l (Stahl et *al.*, 1997). Metabolite levels were not measured. This infant had recently presented with thrombocytopenia and anaemia, which did not resolve until breast-feeding was stopped one month later. No other explanation for the haematological disturbances was found. It is known that valproic acid may cause a variety of blood cell disorders, including bone marrow toxicity. Thrombocytopenia associated with valproic acid may be immunologic in origin, or concentration-dependent (Barr *et al.*, 1982; Gidal *et al.*, 1994). The role of metabolites in the aetiology of this adverse reaction is not known.

Conclusion on valproic acid

Serum levels of valproate in the nursing infant are low and not likely to cause any concentration-dependent adverse effects. However, the possibility of idiosyncratic reactions even to low doses should be observed.

CLONAZEPAM

Milk levels of clonazepam have been reported to be 1 : 3 (Fisher *et al.*, 1985) or 0.37 (Söderman and Matheson, 1988) of the maternal plasma levels. These ratios are slightly higher than those reported for diazepam (0.10–0.20; Erkkola and Kanto, 1972; Dusci *et al.*, 1990), *N*-desmethyldiazepam (0.13; Dusci *et al.*, 1990), oxazepam (0.13; Wretlind, 1987; Dusci *et al.*, 1990), and temazepam (0.14; Dusci *et al.*, 1990).

Respiratory depression was found in two infants who had been exposed to clonazepam during pregnancy, and via breast milk. In one case overt clinical symptoms remained for about 10 days after birth, but excessive periodic breathing was demonstrated for 10 weeks (Fisher *et al.*, 1985). The serum level of clonazepam at 120 hours was 2.9 ng/ml (= 9.1 nmol/l), and on day 14 it was 1 ng/ml (= 3 nmol/l). In the other infant, who was also exposed to phenytoin, signs of respiratory depression lasted for 'at least 14 days' after birth (Söderman and Matheson, 1988). In pooled serum samples from days 2–4 the clonazepam level was 15 nmol/l (= 4.7 ng/ml). In both reported cases, the clinical symptoms were believed to be caused by transplacentally transferred clonazepam, which probably also accounted for the major part of the clonazepam levels in serum.

VIGABATRIN, LAMOTRIGINE, GABAPENTIN, AND FELBAMATE

To date, there seem to be no published data on transfer to breast milk of these new antiepileptic agents. However, it is likely that their levels in breast milk will be lower than in maternal plasma.

Vigabatrin and gabapentin are mainly excreted unchanged in the urine. In infants with fully developed renal function accumulation of these drugs is unlikely.

Lamotrigine is to a large extent glucuronidated via so-called UDP-glucuronosyltransferases. Enzymes of this family glucuronidate many different drugs and endogenous substances, such as bilirubin. In the newborn, the capacity to glucuronidate is not fully developed, but increases gradually during the first months of life. The metabolism of lamotrigine can be induced by phenytoin, phenobarbital, primidone, and carbamazepine, whereas valproic acid decreases the metabolism. It is likely that the infant's capacity to eliminate lamotrigine will be affected by prior or concomitant exposure to any of these drugs.

Felbamate should be avoided during breast-feeding, because of the risk of serious haematological adverse effects, which probably are not directly related to the drug concentrations in plasma.

REFERENCES

Anderson, P.O. (1991). Therapy review. Drug use during breast-feeding. *Clin Pharm* **10**, 594–624.

Atkinson, H.C. and Begg, E.J. (1990). Prediction of drug distribution into human milk from physicochemical characteristics. *Clin Pharmacokinet* **18**, 151–167.

Barr, R.D., Copeland, S.A., Stockwell, M.L., Morris, N. and Kelton, J.C. (1982). Valproic acid and immune thrombocytopenia. *Arch Dis Child* **57**, 681–684.

Bennet, P.N. and the WHO Working Group (1988). *Drugs and Human Lactation.* Elsevier, Amsterdam.

Bertilsson, L. and Tomson, T. (1986). Clinical pharmacokinetics and pharmacological effects of carbamazepine and carbamazepine-10,11-epoxide. *Clin Pharmacokinet* **11**, 177–198.

Bülau, P., Paar, W.D. and von Unruh, G.E. (1988). Pharmacokinetics of oxcarbazepine and 10-hydroxy-carbazepine in the newborn child of an oxcarbazepine-treated mother. *Eur J Clin Pharmacol* **34**, 311–313.

Briggs, G.G., Freeman, R.K. and Yaffe, S.J. (1994). *Drugs in Pregnancy and Lactation, 4th edn.* Williams & Wilkins, Baltimore, MD.

Dusci, L.J., Good, S.M., Hall, R.W. and Ilett, K.F. (1990). Excretion of diazepam and its metabolites in human milk during withdrawal from combination high dose diazepam and oxazepam. *Br J Clin Pharmacol* **29**, 123–126.

Erkkola, R. and Kanto, J. (1972). Diazepam and breast feeding. *Lancet* **i**, 1235–1236.

Finch, E. and Lorber, J. (1954). Methaemoglobinaemia in the newborn: probably due to phenytoin excreted in human milk. *J Obstet Gynaecol Br Emp* **61**, 833.

Fisher, J.B., Edgren, B.E., Mammel, M.C. and Coleman, J.M. (1985). Neonatal apnea associated with maternal clonazepam therapy: a case report. *Obstet Gynecol* **66**, 34S.

Fleishaker, J.C., Desai, N. and McNamara, P.J. (1987). Factors affecting the milk-to-plasma drug concentration ratio in lactating women: physical interactions with protein and fat. *J Pharm Sci* **76**, 189–193.

Frey, B., Schubiger, G. and Musy, J.P. (1990). Transient cholestatic hepatitis in a neonate associated with carbamazepine exposure during pregnancy and breast-feeding. *Eur J Pediatr* **150**, 136–138.

Gidal, B., Spencer, N., Maly, M. *et al.* (1994). Valproate-mediated disturbances of hemostasis: relationship to dose and plasma concentration. *Neurology* **44**, 1418–1422.

Juul, S. (1969). Fenemalforgiftning via modermaelken? *Ugeskr Laeg* **131**, 2257–2258.

Knott, C., Reynolds, F. and Clayden, G. (1987). Infantile spasms on weaning from breast milk containing anticonvulsants. *Lancet* **ii**, 272–273.

Kuhnz, W., Jäger-Roman, E., Rating, D. *et al.* (1983). Carbamazine and carba-mazepine-10,11-epoxide during pregnancy and the postnatal period in epileptic mothers and their nursed infants. Pharmacokinetics and clinical effects. *Pediatr Pharmacol* **3**, 199–208.

Kuhnz, W., Koch, S., Jakob, S., Hartmann, A., Helge, H. and Nau, H. (1984). Ethosuximide in epileptic women during pregnancy and lactation period. Placental transfer, serum concentrations in nursed infants and clinical status. *Br J Clin Pharmacol* **18**, 671–677.

Matheson, I. and Skjaeraasen, J. (1988). Milk concentrations of flupenthixol, nortriptyline and zuclopenthixol and between-breast differences in two patients. *Eur J Pharmacol* **35**, 217–220.

Merlob, P., Mor, N. and Litwin, A. (1992). Transient hepatic dysfunction in an infant of an epileptic mother treated with carbamazepine during pregnancy and breast-feeding. *Ann Pharmacother* **26**, 1563–1565.

Meyer, F.P., Quednow, B., Potrafik, A. and Walther, H. (1988). Zur Pharmacokinetik von Antiepileptika in der Perinatalperiode. *Zent bl Gynäkol* **110**, 1195–1205.

Nau, H., Rating, D., Koch, S., Häuser, I. and Helge, H. (1981). Valproic acid and its metabolites: placental transfer, neonatal pharmacokinetics, transfer via mother's milk and clinical status in neonates of epileptic mothers. *J Pharmacol Exp Ther* **219**, 768–777.

Nau, H., Kuhnz, W., Egger, H.-J., Rating, D. and Helge, H. (1982). Anticonvulsants during pregnancy and lactation: transplacental, maternal and neonatal pharma-cokinetics. *Clin Pharmacokinet* **7**, 508–543.

Philbert, A., Pedersen, B. and Dam, M. (1985). Concentration of valproate during pregnancy, in the newborn and in breast milk. *Acta Neurol Scand* **72**, 460–463.

Pynnönen, S., Kanto, J., Sillanpää, M. and Erkkola, R. (1977). Carbamazepine: placental transport, tissue concentrations in foetus and newborn, and level in milk. *Acta Pharmacol Toxicol* **41**, 244–253.

Rane, A. and Tunell, R. (1981). Ethosuximide in human milk and in plasma of a mother and her nursed infant. *Br J Clin Pharmacol* **12**, 855–858.

Rane, A., Garle, M., Borgå, O. and Sjöqvist, F. (1974). Plasma disappearance of transplacentally transferred diphenylhydantoin in the newborn: studies by mass fragmentography. *Clin Pharmacol Ther* **15**, 39–45.

Söderman, P. and Rane, A. (1986). *Ethosuximide and nursing (Abstract no. 518).* Third World Conference on Clinical Pharmacology and Therapeutics, Stockholm, 1986.

Söderman, P. and Matheson, I. (1988). Clonazepam in breast milk. *Eur J Pediatr* **147**, 212–213.

Söderman, P., Elwin, C.-E., Lidén, A. and Voss, H. (1986). Amning vid behandling med primidon. Abstract presented at Svenska Läkarsällskapets Riksstämma, Stockholm, 1986.

Stahl, M.M.S., Neiderud, J. and Vinge, E. (1997). Thrombocytopenic purpura and anaemia in a suckling whose mother was treated with valproic acid. *J Pediatr* (in press).

Steen, B., Rane, A., Lönnerholm, G., Falk, O., Elwin, C.-E. and Sjöqvist, F. (1982). Phenytoin excretion in human breast milk and plasma levels in nursed infants. *Ther Drug Monit* **4**, 331–334.

Stricker, B.H.Ch. (1992). *Drug-Induced Hepatic Injury, 2nd edn. Drug-Induced Disorders, Vol. 5* (Series Editor: M.N.G. Dukes). Elsevier, Amsterdam, pp. 157–159.

Tomson, T. and Villén, T. (1994). Ethosuximide enantiomers in pregnancy and lactation. *Ther Drug Monit* **16**, 621–623.

Tyson, R.M., Shrader, E.A. and Perlman, H.N. (1938). Drugs transmitted through breast-milk. II. Barbiturates. *J Pediatr* **13**, 86–90.

Wretlind, M. (1987). Excretion of oxazepam in breast milk. *Eur J Clin Pharmacol* **33**, 209–210.

Epilepsy and Pregnancy
Edited by T. Tomson, L. Gram, M. Sillanpää and S.I. Johannessen
© 1997 Wrightson Biomedical Publishing Ltd

10

Complications During Pregnancy and Delivery

ANNE SABERS

Department of Neurology, State University Hospital, Copenhagen, Denmark

INTRODUCTION

Women with epilepsy have been described as having more complications during pregnancy and delivery than women in general (Bjerkedal and Bahna, 1973). The complications may adversely affect the course and outcome of pregnancy with respect to abortions, intrauterine fetal growth retardation, development of congenital malformations, perinatal asphyxia and survival of the fetus. Maternal complications include vaginal bleeding, preeclampsia, prolonged labour and surgical delivery as well as a risk of increased seizure frequency during the pregnancy.

At least three factors, genetic aspects, seizures themselves, exposure to antiepileptic drugs, and combinations of these factors, separate women with epilepsy from women without epilepsy and may, therefore, contribute to the increased risk of complications in the epilepsy group.

However, the complication rate varies greatly among the studies reported in the literature and data are often conflicting.

This chapter reviews the literature on fetal and maternal complications. Teratogenic aspects and the effect of pregnancy on maternal epilepsy are discussed elsewhere. Some of the results of our own retrospective study on the outcome of pregnancy in 151 patients with epilepsy (not yet published) are presented (Table 1).

FETAL COMPLICATIONS

Spontaneous abortion

The exact number of spontaneous abortions is difficult to estimate even in carefully controlled studies as some abortions may have passed unrecognized

Table 1. Neonatal, maternal and obstetric outcome in 151 pregnancies of women with epilepsy compared with 38 983 deliveries in the background population. A retrospective study at Hvidovre Hospital, Denmark, 1978–1992.

		Women with epilepsy		95% CI	Background population	
		n	%		n	%
Sex distribution: female		72	48	(40.51–56.97)	18 751	48
	male	79	52	(43.69–60.14)	20 460	51
Birthweight	< 2500 g	7	5	(1.88–9.43)	2 699	7
	> 4500 g	7	5	(1.88–9.43)	1 458	4
Preeclampsia		12	8*	(4.2–13.6)	1 247	3
Preterm births		7	5	(1.9–9.4)	2 699	7
Induction of labour		42	28*	(21.03–35.93)	3 606	9
Vacuum extraction		23	15	(9.99–22.14)	4 938	13
Caesarean section		18	12	(7.28–18.33)	4 181	11
Perinatal deaths		2	1.3	(0.2–4.7)	181	0.5

*Significant

or before antenatal booking. However, the majority of reports indicate that spontaneous abortions are not more common in women with epilepsy than in the general population (Andermann *et al.*, 1982; Annegers *et al.*, 1988; Hunter and Allen, 1990).

Intrauterine growth retardation

Low birthweight for gestational age is more frequent in infants of women with epilepsy than controls (Bjerkedal and Bahna, 1973; Andermann *et al.*, 1982; Yerby *et al.*, 1985; Akhtar and Millac, 1987; Mastroiacovo *et al.*, 1988; Martin and Millac, 1993). Mastroiacovo *et al.* (1988) observed an increased occurrence of intrauterine growth retardation amongst infants of women with epilepsy, even in untreated women, which suggests a maternal disease effect. When specific monotherapies were taken into account, only exposure of phenobarbitone was associated with reduced birthweight (Mastroiacovo *et al.*, 1988). In a study comparing the outcomes of pregnancy in two periods, 1977 to 1981 and 1987 to 1991 (Martin and Millac, 1993), the percentages of low birthweight infants were constant and always higher among infants of women with epilepsy (10.6% and 9.4%, respectively) than in controls during the two periods (8.5% and 6.7%, respectively). There was a marked change in anticonvulsant prescribing away from phenobarbitone and phenytoin towards carbamazepine and sodium valproate in the second period; however, more patients were treated with polytherapy in the second period. In contrast with these findings, low birthweight was not observed in four prospective studies (Hiilesmaa *et al.*, 1985; Hunter and Allen, 1990; Tanganelli and Regesta, 1992; Steegers-Theunissen *et al.*, 1994). In these studies, the majority of patients were monitored frequently during pregnancy and mainly kept on low to moderate doses of a single antiepileptic drug.

A slight, but significant, smaller head circumference among infants born to mothers with epilepsy has been reported by several authors (Ogawa et al., 1982; Neri et al., 1983; Mastroiacovo et al., 1988; Steegers-Theunissen et al., 1994) whereas neonatal birth length appears not to be affected in newborns of women with epilepsy (Neri et al., 1983; Mastroiacovo et al., 1988; Steegers-Theunissen et al., 1994).

Use of antiepileptic drugs seems to have no effect on intrauterine fetal heart rate and motility (van Geijn et al., 1986; Swartjes et al., 1992).

Placental weights (Ogawa et al., 1982), placental morphology and growth factor receptors (Eeg-Olofsson et al., 1990) are not affected by antiepileptic drug exposure.

Perinatal asphyxia and infant mortality

Low Apgar scores and development of asphyxia have been found in a larger proportion of infants of women with epilepsy than in controls and it is suggested that these infants might be more vulnerable due to the effect of antiepileptic medication (Yerby et al., 1985). In a study of sodium valproate monotherapy on pregnancy outcome almost half of the infants were distressed during labour as against 9% in controls, and 28% had low Apgar scores versus 5.5% among controls (Jäger-Roman et al., 1986). Hiilesmaa et al. (1985) found that early heart decelerations of the fetus were more frequent among women with epilepsy during labour; however, asphyxia was not significantly increased in newborns of women with epilepsy than in matched controls .This is in agreement with the study by Neri et al. (1983) who found no association between asphyxia and maternal epilepsy or antiepileptic drug treatment. Transient fetal asphyxia can be caused by a generalized tonic-clonic seizure during labour (Teramo et al., 1979).

Perinatal mortality in infants of women with epilepsy has been found to be two to three times higher than in the general population in several both retrospective and prospective studies (Bjerkedal and Bahna, 1973; Andermann et al., 1982; Hiilesmaa et al., 1985; Källen, 1986; Akhtar and Millac, 1987; Martin and Millac, 1993). Martin and Millac (1993) found a fall in perinatal mortality rate when outcomes of pregnancies were compared in two periods, from 1977 to 1981 and from 1987 to 1991, from 4.7% to 2.1%, respectively. The mortality rate, however, was constantly two to three times that of the respective control groups which, therefore, reflects better perinatal care during recent years in general rather than an effect of changed antiepileptic prescription. Andermann et al. (1982) found that perinatal deaths occurred more frequently in women with epilepsy than in spouses of men with epilepsy (6.2% versus 1.0%). These data suggest that genetic factors may be of minor importance in the aetiology of perinatal deaths. However, a genetic predisposing link might exist between maternal epilepsy and fetal death, such as suggested for certain malformations (Lindhout and Omtzigt, 1992).

MATERNAL COMPLICATIONS

Vaginal bleeding

The amount of blood lost at delivery has been described as higher among women with epilepsy than among control mothers (Bjerkedal and Bahna, 1973; Egenaes, 1982). Ablatio placentae, vitamin K deficiency, and hypotonic uterine activity have been claimed as the main important causes of the vaginal bleeding observed (Egenaes, 1982). Other authors report no significant differences in the incidence of vaginal bleeding among women taking antiepileptic drugs compared with controls (Andermann et al., 1982; Ogawa et al., 1982; Hiilesmaa et al., 1985; Tanganelli and Regesta, 1992). It is possible, but not clearly described in recent studies, that maternal coagulation deficiencies have been prevented by prophylactic vitamin K supplement given during the last month of pregnancy.

Toxaemia

Preeclampsia is twice as frequent in women with epilepsy compared with controls in some studies (Bjerkedal and Bahna, 1973; Janz and Beck-Mannagetta, 1982; Yerby et al., 1985). We found significant increased incidence of preeclampsia among women with epilepsy (Table 1). Other studies found no differences between the frequency of preeclampsia in women with epilepsy and women without epilepsy (Andermann et al., 1982; Egenaes, 1982; Tanganelli and Regesta, 1992). However, more serious cases of preeclampsia appeared to be slightly more frequent in women with epilepsy than in controls (Egenaes, 1982).

Preterm and prolonged labour

Neither preterm labour (Hiilesmaa et al., 1985; Akhtar and Millac, 1987; Tanganelli and Regesta, 1992) nor prolonged labour lasting more than 24 hours seem to occur more frequently in women with epilepsy than in controls (Andermann et al., 1982; Ogawa et al., 1982).

Induction of labour

Induction of labour is used more frequently in women with epilepsy (Bjerkedal and Bahna, 1973; Andermann et al., 1982; Egenaes, 1982; Yerby *et al.*, 1985). Labour is induced 4.3 times as often in women with epilepsy compared with controls (Yerby *et al.*, 1985). Whether the high number of inductions is a result of an actual increased complication rate is debated. Deliveries among women with epilepsy may be more probably planned to take place at the most convenient hour of the day, when the best-trained staff are on duty (Egenaes, 1982). The duration of labour may more often be shortened with the aim of avoiding stress and the tiring of the woman with epilepsy. In our study, induction of labour was significantly more frequent in women with epilepsy (Table 1). The reasons for the induction were preeclampsia, prolonged labour or fetal distress, in most cases.

Instrumental delivery

Bjerkedal and Bahna (1973) reported a 1.89% incidence of abnormal presentation in patients with epilepsy compared with 0.87% in controls. The need for forceps or vacuum extraction and the rate of delivery by caesarean section in this study were more than twice as frequent in women with epilepsy than in controls. Although increased rates of caesarean sections have been confirmed by several other authors (Vert *et al.*, 1979; Bossi *et al.*, 1980; Andermann *et al.*, 1982; Egenaes, 1982; Yerby *et al.*, 1985), there is no evidence that this is a result of obstetric complications. There is possibly a tendency for obstetricians to interfere more frequently in the deliveries of women with epilepsy because of anxiety in handling this group of patients (Hiilesmaa *et al.*, 1985). In accordance with our study (Table 1) most recent studies demonstrate no increased frequency of surgical or instrumental deliveries in women with epilepsy compared with controls (Hiilesmaa *et al.*, 1985; Akhtar and Millac, 1987; Hunter and Allen, 1990; Tanganelli and Regesta, 1992).

CONCLUSIONS

This review of the literature demonstrates that the complication rate during pregnancy and delivery in women with epilepsy varies greatly among the studies and data are often conflicting. Many studies are retrospective or based on registries. At least some of the complications which are more frequently reported in women with epilepsy than in the general population may depend on reporting biases as a result of increased attention to this group of pregnant patients; a possible anxiety among obstetricians handling women with epilepsy may explain some of the findings.

It is prudent that treatment for women with epilepsy be provided at obstetric centres with the experience and the resources to attend to the specific problems that may occur. Given the advantages of modern medical management, most women with epilepsy can be assured of a good obstetric and neonatal outcome.

REFERENCES

Akhtar, N. and Millac, P. (1987). Epilepsy and pregnancy: a study of 188 pregnancies in 92 patients. *Br J Clin Pract* **41**, 862–864.

Andermann, E., Dansky, L. and Kinch, R.A. (1982). Complications of pregnancy, labour and delivery in epileptic women. In: Janz, D., Dam, M., Richens, A., Bossi, L., Helge, H. and Schmidt, D. (Eds), *Epilepsy, Pregnancy, and the Child*. Raven Press, New York, pp. 61–74.

Annegers, J.F., Baumgartner, K.B., Hauser, W.A. and Kurland, L.T. (1988). Epilepsy, antiepileptic drugs, and the risk of spontaneous abortion. *Epilepsia* **29**, 451–458.

Bjerkedal, T. and Bahna, S.L. (1973). The course and outcome of pregnancy in women with epilepsy. *Acta Obstet Gynecol Scand* **52**, 245–248.

Bossi, L., Assael, B.M., Avanzini, G. *et al.* (1980). Plasma levels and clinical effects of antiepileptic drugs in pregnant epileptic patients and their newborns. In: Johannessen, S.I., Morselli, P.L., Pippenger, C.E., Richens, A., Schmidt, D. and Meinardi, H. (Eds), *Antiepileptic Therapy: Advances in Drug Monitoring*. Raven Press, New York, pp. 9–18.

Eeg-Olofsson, O., Chen, M.F., Andermann, E., Dansky, L., Guyda, H.J. and Kinch, R.A.H. (1990). Evaluation of placental morphology and growth factor receptors in women receiving antiepileptic drugs: a pilot study. *Epilepsia* **31**, 446–452.

Egenaes, J. (1982). Outcome of pregnancy in women with epilepsy — Norway, 1967 to 1978. In: Janz, D., Dam, M., Richens, A., Bossi, L., Helge, H. and Schmidt, D. (Eds), *Epilepsy, Pregnancy and the Child*. Raven Press, New York, pp. 81–55.

Hiilesmaa, V.K., Bardy, A. and Teramo, K. (1985). Obstetric outcome in women with epilepsy. *Am J Obstet Gynecol* **152**, 499–504.

Hunter, R.W. and Allen, E.M. (1990). The course and outcome of pregnancy in women with epilepsy – a 6-year prospective study. *J Obstet Gynecol* **10**, 483–491.

Janz, D. and Beck-Mannagetta, G. (1982). Complications of pregnancy in women with epilepsy: a retrospective study. In: Janz, D., Dam, M., Richens, A., Bossi, L., Helge, H. and Schmidt, D. (Eds), *Epilepsy, Pregnancy, and the Child*. Raven Press, New York, pp. 103–105.

Jäger-Roman, E., Deichl, A., Jakob, S. *et al.* (1986). Fetal growth, major malformations, and minor anomalies in infants born to women receiving valproic acid. *J Pediatr* **108**, 997–1004.

Källen, B. (1986). A register study of maternal epilepsy and delivery outcome with special reference to drug use. *Acta Neurol Scand* **73**, 253–259.

Lindhout, D. and Omtzigt, J.G.C. (1992). Pregnancy and the risk of teratogenicity. *Epilepsia* **33** (suppl 4), 41–48.

Martin, P.J. and Millac, P.A.H. (1993). Pregnancy, epilepsy, management and outcome: a 10-year prospective study. *Seizure* **2**, 227–280.

Mastroiacovo, P., Bertollini, R. and Licata, D. (1988). Fetal growth in the offspring of epileptic women: results of an Italian multicentric cohort study. *Acta Neurol Scand* **78**, 110–114.

Neri, A., Heifez, L., Nitke, S. and Ovadia, J. (1983). Neonatal outcome in infants of epileptic mothers. *Eur J Obstet Gynecol Reprod Biol* **16**, 263–268.

Ogawa, Y., Nomura, Y., Kaneko, S., Suzuki, K. and Sato, T. (1982). Insidious effect of antiepileptic drugs in the perinatal period. In: Janz, D., Dam, M., Richens, A., Bossi, L., Helge, H. and Schmidt, D. (Eds), *Epilepsy, Pregnancy, and the Child.* Raven Press, New York, pp. 197–202.

Steegers-Theunissen, R.P.M., Reiner, O.W., Borm, G.F. *et al.* (1994). Factors influencing the risk of abnormal pregnancy outcome in epileptic women: a multicenter prospective study. *Epilepsy Res* **18**, 261–269.

Swartjes, J.M., van Geijn, H.P., Meinardi, H., van Woerden, E.E. and Mantel, R. (1992). Fetal motility and chronic exposure to antiepileptic drugs. *Eur J Obstet Gynecol Reprod Biol* **45**, 37–45.

Tanganelli, P. and Regesta, G. (1992). Epilepsy, pregnancy, and major birth anomalies: an Italian prospective, controlled study. *Neurology* **42** (suppl 5), 89–93.

Teramo, K., Hiilesmaa, V., Bardy, A. and Saarikoski, S. (1979). Fetal heart rate during a maternal grand mal epileptic seizure. *J Perinat Med* **7**, 3–6.

van Geijn, H.P., Swartjes, J.M., van Woerden, E.E., Caron, F.J.M., Brons, J.T.J. and Arts, N.F.T. (1986). Fetal behavioural states in epileptic pregnancies. *Eur J Obstet Gynecol Reprod Biol* **21**, 309–314.

Vert, P., André, M. and Deblay, M.F. (1979). Infants of epileptic mothers. In: Stern, L. (Ed.), *Intensive Care in Newborns, II.* Masson, New York, pp. 347–360.

Yerby, M., Koepsell, T. and Daling, J. (1985). Pregnancy complications and outcomes in a cohort of women with epilepsy. *Epilepsy* **26**, 631–635.

Epilepsy and Pregnancy
Edited by T. Tomson, L. Gram, M. Sillanpää and S.I. Johannessen
© 1997 Wrightson Biomedical Publishing Ltd

11

Seizure Control During Pregnancy and Delivery

TORBJÖRN TOMSON
Department of Clinical Neuroscience, Karolinska Hospital, Stockholm, Sweden

INTRODUCTION

The challenge of pharmacotherapy of epilepsy is to balance the benefits of drug therapy in terms of reducing the risk of seizures against the risk of side-effects of antiepileptic drugs. This balance is even more delicate when the woman with epilepsy becomes pregnant. In this situation, any possible effects of both drugs and seizures on the fetus also need to be taken into account. The situation constitutes a therapeutic dilemma since, on the one hand, antiepileptic drugs are teratogenic and, on the other, uncontrolled seizures may be hazardous to the fetus (see Chapter 13) as well as to the pregnant woman. Most physicians would agree that, in the interest of both the fetus and the mother, antiepileptic drugs are indicated during pregnancy when necessary for the prevention of tonic-clonic seizures. The treatment should aim at total control of such seizures during pregnancy. To achieve this, it is important to know how seizure control may be affected by pregnancy. What is the risk of an increase in seizure frequency? When, during pregnancy, is such a change most likely to occur? Can pregnancy induce a lasting deterioration in seizure control? Which risk factors may be identified and which are the mechanisms behind a possible alteration in seizure control? Answers to these questions are needed to optimize drug therapy during pregnancy, and are furthermore valuable for a professional pre-pregnancy counselling. These questions and related issues will be discussed in the present review. This chapter will focus on recent research. For a comprehensive review of the topic from 1884 to 1980, see Schmidt (1982).

THE EFFECT OF PREGNANCY ON EPILEPSY – METHODOLOGICAL ASPECTS

The design of a study of epilepsy during pregnancy must depend on the specific question to be answered. In order to evaluate the effect of pregnancy on seizure propensity, seizure frequency in pregnant women with epilepsy should be compared with that of a control group, such as adequately matched nonpregnant epileptic women. The author is not aware of any such study.

Most investigators have, as an alternative, used the pregnant epileptic woman as her own control, comparing seizure frequency during pregnancy with that of a pregestational baseline period in the same individual. This approach highlights another fundamental methodological issue: the importance of a prospective design. Most early reports, and some more recent (Wilhelm *et al.*, 1990; Lander and Eadie, 1991) appear to be based on retrospective reviews of cohorts of pregnant epileptic women. The more recent prospective studies, however, are prospective only during pregnancy. Seizure control during the pregestational reference period is assessed in retrospect through patient recall or case records. Hence, the information on occurrence of seizures is more reliable during pregnancy than during the retrospective control period. The most probable consequence of this is an underestimation of seizure frequency before pregnancy.

Another confounding factor related to this design is that the management of the patient will be different during pregnancy compared with the reference period. The prospective protocol generally prescribes frequent clinical appointments with drug level monitoring at regular intervals during pregnancy, which most probably enhance compliance and thus affect seizure control (Cramer *et al.*, 1990). The readiness to adjust drug dosages may also be quite different, and also the foundation for such decisions, considering the drug level monitoring policy of most prospective protocols. A consequence may be an underestimation of a possible detrimental effect of pregnancy on seizure control.

At best, these prospective studies with retrospective controls provide information on seizure control during gestation in a specific patient population, managed according to the therapeutic principles of that study protocol. Such information is meaningful only if the management of the patients is described and, furthermore, criteria for changes in drug therapy are given, so that this may be replicated. Surprisingly, such information is often lacking (Wilhelm *et al.*, 1990; Tanganelli and Regesta, 1992).

From studies where such criteria are accounted for, it is obvious that differences in treatment policies are pronounced. As an example, doses of antiepileptic drugs were adjusted during pregnancy in anything from 16% (Tomson *et al.*, 1994) to 80% (Lander and Eadie, 1991) of the cases. Criteria for dose adjustments, if stated, ranged from 'when there is a change in drug levels' (Lander and Eadie, 1991) to 'only when necessary to combat increased seizure frequency' (Bardy, 1987; Gjerde *et al.*, 1988; Tomson *et al.*, 1994).

Seizure control during pregnancy may also be compared with a *postgestational* reference period, thus avoiding the drawbacks of a retrospective pregestational baseline (Canger *et al.*, 1982). However, seizure control after delivery is likely to be affected by sleep deprivation and other factors related to the new family situation. In addition, a lasting deterioration in seizure control induced by pregnancy may imply a carry-over effect of pregnancy on the reference period.

A further methodological issue of concern is related to the definition of the major outcome measures in different studies. In general, this is expressed as an increase, decrease or no change in seizure frequency during pregnancy, compared with the reference period. However, the criteria for these categories vary markedly between studies and are sometimes not given (Knight and Rhind, 1975; Lander and Eadie, 1991). Some authors regard an increase or decrease in seizure frequency of more than 15% as indicating a change (Fröscher et al., 1991); others require a variation greater than 200% (Wilhelm et al., 1990). It goes without saying that it is difficult to compare studies with such divergent criteria for outcome measures. Another common approach is to classify patients into different categories according to seizure frequency during the nine pregestational months. The change in seizure frequency is then defined as a movement from one frequency category to another (Canger et al., 1982; Otani, 1985; Tomson et al., 1994).

A key question is to what extent the results of previous studies allow conclusions to be drawn concerning seizure control in the general population of pregnant women with epilepsy. This external validity of the results depends on the degree of patient selection in the studies. In this respect, it is a matter of concern that most reports come from epilepsy centres, presumably with a patient selection biased towards more severe epilepsy (Canger et al., 1982; Schmidt et al., 1982, 1983; Remillard et al., 1982). This reduces the validity of these studies, particularly since severe epilepsy may be related to a higher risk of deterioration in seizure control during pregnancy. The fact that a large proportion of patients is excluded from the analysis in some studies further complicates their interpretation (Remillard et al., 1982; Canger et al., 1982). In general, the selection process is not reported and estimates of the representativeness of the study population are rare. There are only a few reports which are more or less population-based (Bardy, 1987; Gjerde et al., 1988; Tomson et al., 1994). In the prospective studies from Helsinki and Stockholm, it was estimated that 75–80% of all women with epilepsy who were pregnant during the study periods were included in the respective study populations. This therefore indicates that results from these studies may be taken as being representative for the population of pregnant epileptic women as a whole.

THE WOMAN WITH EPILEPSY WHO BECOMES PREGNANT

Women with epilepsy who become pregnant may for several reasons be different from the general epilepsy population. Fertility is decreased among patients with severe epilepsy and these patients are also less likely to form relationships.

In early reports and some recent publications from epilepsy centres, the study populations are dominated by women with partial seizures and poor seizure control (Canger *et al.*, 1982; Remillard *et al.*, 1982; Otani, 1985; Wilhelm *et al.*, 1990). In the more recent population-based studies of less selected patients, it can be found that 55–65% of the pregnant women had primary generalized epilepsy (Bardy, 1987; Tanganelli and Regesta, 1992; Tomson *et al.*, 1994), which is a somewhat higher proportion than in the general adult epilepsy population (Forsgren, 1992). Furthermore, as many as 49–65% of the patients in these studies were seizure-free before pregnancy (Otani, 1985; Bardy, 1987; Gjerde *et al.*, 1988; Tomson *et al.*, 1994). Thus, patients with primary generalized epilepsy and good seizure control seem to be overrepresented among epileptic women who become pregnant. This preponderance of easy-to-treat epilepsies is not surprising, but it should be borne in mind when treatment strategies are discussed. As an example, the therapeutic ranges of antiepileptic drug levels often referred to are based on experience from more severe epilepsies.

SEIZURE ONSET DURING PREGNANCY

This chapter is primarily focused on the effect of pregnancy on seizure control in patients with established epilepsy. Some women, however, may experience the onset of a seizure disorder during pregnancy. The possibility of eclampsia needs to be excluded if seizures occur for the first time in the last 20 weeks of pregnancy.

Seizures unrelated to eclampsia may also occur for the first time during pregnancy. Schmidt (1982) found that, in reports of pregnant women with epilepsy, epilepsy had begun during pregnancy in 13% of cases. He concluded that the incidence of epilepsy among pregnant women was within the expected range for the general population. Knight and Rhind (1975), in their study of 153 pregnancies, found that epilepsy occurred for the first time during pregnancy in 11% of the pregnancies; Lander and Eadie (1991) reported *de novo* seizures in five of 105 pregnancies.

Although the incidence of epilepsy does not appear to be markedly increased during pregnancy, some patients have seizures exclusively during pregnancy. Such strictly gestational seizures constitute a quarter to one-third of all cases of new-onset epilepsy during pregnancy (Schmidt, 1982; Dalessio, 1985).

SEIZURE CONTROL DURING PREGNANCY

Reports of the effect of pregnancy on epilepsy have been published for more than a century (Nerlinger, 1889). Schmidt (1982) reviewed the 2165 pregnancies in published reports up till 1980 and concluded that seizure frequency increased in 24%, decreased in 23%, and remained unchanged in 53% of

Table 1. Seizure control in pregnancy.

Author, year	Study design/ population	No. of pregnancies	Seizure-free before pregnancy (%)	Seizure frequency during pregnancy		
				Increased (%)	Unchanged (%)	Decreased (%)
Canger et al., 1982	Prospective/selected	34	N/A	41	50	9
Schmidt et al., 1982	Prospective/selected	33	48	8	87	5
Remillard et al., 1982	Prospective/selected	56	55	46	50	4
Schmidt et al., 1983	Prospective/selected	136	N/A	37	50	13
Otani, 1985	Prospective/unclear	110	65	23	70	7
Bardy, 1987	Prospective/population based	154	49	32	54	14
Gjerde et al., 1988	Prospective/population-based	78	58	17	67	17
Wilhelm et al., 1990	Retrospective/selected	98	54	24	63	6
Lander and Eadie, 1991	Retrospective/selected	134	51	25	65	8
Lopes-Cendes et al., 1992	Prospective/unclear	254	N/A	17	N/A	N/A
Tanganelli and Regesta, 1992	Prospective/selected	138	39	17	80	3
Tomson et al., 1994	Prospective/population-based	93	55	15	61	24

N/A, data not available.

cases. These conclusions were drawn from predominantly retrospective studies with all the inherent limitations discussed above.

The outcome of subsequent studies (summarized in Table 1) reveals wide variation in their results. The percentage of patients experiencing an increase in seizure frequency during pregnancy ranges from 8% to 46%. However, taken together, the results of the studies reported in Table 1 are similar to those of the early studies, despite differences in patient populations, study design, criteria for outcome measures, and in therapeutic strategies. Twenty to twenty-five per cent of the patients deteriorate in seizure control during gestation regardless of whether the evaluation is confined to more recent population-based studies, prospective studies since 1985, or all studies after 1982. This consistency in results over the decades, despite a presumed advance in medical care, can have several explanations, as discussed above. A further reason may be a seemingly paradoxical consequence of the inclusion of more patients with well-controlled epilepsy in recent population-based studies. Patients with full pregestational seizure control can, at best, maintain the seizure control during pregnancy, but not improve. Hence, the larger the proportion of patients with well controlled epilepsy in a study, the smaller the chance that patients will improve during pregnancy. One may, however, conclude from these studies that, with the management offered to pregnant women with epilepsy, the majority can expect to have at least as good a seizure control during pregnancy as before.

A matter of special concern is status epilepticus during pregnancy, considering the associated risk to both the pregnant women and the fetus (Philbert and Dam, 1982; Sabers and Dam, 1990). In his review, Schmidt (1982) concluded that status epilepticus occurred in fewer than 1% of all pregnancies of epileptic women, and that status thus does not seem to occur more frequently during pregnancy than at other times of life. Subsequent reports seem to corroborate this statement (see Table 2).

Even though only a minority of patients deteriorate in seizure control it is of importance *when* during pregnancy this is most likely to occur. However, available data are conflicting. Knight and Rhind (1975) reported that the risk of an increase in seizure frequency was highest during the first trimester. This is confirmed by Canger *et al.* (1982). In 11 out of 14 patients who experienced an increase in seizure frequency in their study, the increase occurred in the first or at the beginning of the second trimester. This is further supported by results of the extended material in the collaborative study from Berlin and Milan (Schmidt *et al.*, 1983). The authors conclude that, in most pregnancies with an increase in seizure frequency, it begins in the first trimester, while it is lowest in the third. In contrast, however, Remillard *et al.* (1982) found that the risk of seizure increase was highest during the third trimester. Furthermore, in the prospective population-based Helsinki study there was a tendency for both convulsive seizures and complex partial seizures to increase towards the end of pregnancy rather than during the first two trimesters

Table 2. Status epilepticus in pregnancy.

Author	Number of pregnancies	Cases of status epilepticus
Canger et al., 1982	34	0
Schmidt et al., 1982	33	1
Remillard et al., 1982	56	2
Otani, 1985	110	1
Bardy, 1987	154	0
Gjerde et al., 1988	78	1
Wilhelm et al., 1990	98	1
Tanganelli and Regesta, 1992	138	0
Tomson et al., 1994	93	1

(Bardy, 1987). This result is also found in another population-based study where in fact seizure control seemed to be slightly improved during the first trimester, as compared with the pre-pregnancy period (Tomson et al., 1994). Obviously, there is no consensus regarding which period of pregnancy carries the highest risk of deterioration in seizure control. Depending on the mechanisms behind the loss of seizure control, the conflicting results may in part be explained by differences between the studies with respect to pre-pregnancy counselling and management during pregnancy.

Although unclear whether any trimester is associated with a higher risk of seizure increase, it seems undisputed that the period of labour and delivery carries a particular risk of seizure occurrence. According to Schmidt et al. (1982), generalized tonic-clonic seizures relapsed or increased during or shortly after delivery in four out of 38 cases (11%). In two out of 110 pregnancies in the study of Otani (1985), seizures occurred during or immediately after delivery. Wilhelm and co-workers (1990) reported that four out of 98 women had intrapartum seizures, including one who developed status epilepticus. In addition, five pregnancies were complicated by seizures following delivery, but no details are given. The most elaborate analysis is made by Bardy (1987). In his Helsinki study, seizures occurred during delivery, or within 24 hours from onset of labour, in 10 out of 154 cases. This incidence was estimated to be ninefold greater than the average incidence during pregnancy. However, in another prospective study of 138 pregnancies, Tanganelli and Regesta (1992) observed no seizures during labour. Taking these five studies together, 25 out of 538 cases (5%) had seizures during labour, delivery, or immediately thereafter.

SEIZURE CONTROL AFTER PREGNANCY

A critical question, not least for pre-pregnancy counselling, is whether pregnancy implies a significant risk of deterioration in seizure control outlasting pregnancy. Or can patients who experience seizure exacerbation during pregnancy expect to regain their pregestational seizure control after pregnancy? This important issue has been addressed by some investigators. Knight and Rhind (1975), for example, reported an increased number of seizures in 38 out of 100 pregnancies in patients with idiopathic epilepsy. Three out of the 38 cases were found to have a permanent deterioration long after pregnancy. However, this was balanced by two cases with a lasting improvement dating from pregnancy. Canger *et al.* (1982) evaluated the course of epilepsy after delivery in 11 of the 17 patients who had had a change in seizure frequency during pregnancy. They found that seizure frequency reverted to pregestational levels after pregnancy in all but one case. During a two-year postgestational follow-up of this patient the only seizure manifestation was a single grand mal status five months postpartum. Fröscher and co-workers (1991) made a nine-month follow-up postpartum of 39 pregnancies. Of those who had had an increased seizure frequency during pregnancy, 88% with generalized tonic-clonic seizures and 83% with complex partial seizures returned to normal seizure control during the nine months postpartum. In the prospective Italian study by Tanganelli and Regesta (1992), seizure frequency reverted to pre-pregnancy levels during puerperium in all but two women of the 24 whose seizure control had deteriorated during pregnancy. These fairly consistent results stand in contrast to a recent report by Drislane (1994), based on a retrospective case-record review. He found that five out of 31 patients who were referred to an epilepsy centre *after* pregnancy had major and prolonged deterioration in their epilepsy following pregnancy. The exacerbations are reported to have persisted for many years. All five patients had partial seizures and the author speculates on the role of elevation of oestrogen levels during pregnancy in the long-lasting deterioration. The contrast between this report and other studies should be seen in the light of the referral pattern and retrospective nature of the Drislane study. Prospective studies strongly suggest that protracted worsening of epilepsy associated with pregnancy is uncommon. In fact it is so rare that it may well be unrelated to pregnancy and rather an expression of the unstable nature of epilepsy as such.

CLINICAL FACTORS RELATED TO ALTERED SEIZURE CONTROL

Though the epilepsy obviously seems to be unaffected by pregnancy in the majority of patients, attempts have been made to identify the patient at risk for an increase in seizures during gestation. There are a number of large prospective studies, some of which are population-based, where no clinical features predicting a change in seizure control have been identified (Schmidt *et al.*, 1982; Schmidt *et al.*, 1983; Bardy, 1987; Gjerde *et al.*, 1988). However, in many studies two clinical characteristics of the patient's epilepsy have emerged as risk factors for an increase in seizure frequency during pregnancy. First, partial or localization-related epilepsy as opposed to primary generalized epilepsy has frequently been associated with a higher risk of deterioration (Canger *et al.*, 1982; Remillard *et al.*, 1982; Otani, 1985; Fröscher *et al.*, 1991; Tanganelli and Regesta, 1992; Lopes-Cendes *et al.*, 1992; Tomson *et al.*, 1994). Secondly, many studies report that patients with good seizure control before pregnancy are less likely to deteriorate than patients with a high seizure frequency (Knight and Rhind, 1975; Remillard *et al.*, 1982; Wilhelm *et al.*, 1990; Lander and Eadie, 1991; Lopes-Cendes *et al.*, 1992). An intriguing observation in the large study by Lopes-Cendes *et al.* (1992) was that the most significant risk factor was failure to have pre-pregnancy counselling. This observation corresponds well with the favourable outcomes found in a population with a comparatively high proportion of patients undertaking pre-pregnancy counselling (Tomson *et al.*, 1994).

MECHANISMS BEHIND LOSS OF SEIZURE CONTROL

Several factors may contribute to an altered seizure frequency during pregnancy. Pregnancy-induced changes in the kinetics of antiepileptic drugs is one factor that has been given much attention (see Chapter 7). However, most studies have failed to demonstrate a relationship between changes in serum levels of antiepileptic drugs and seizure control. This may in part be explained by the fact that unbound drug levels tend to decrease much less than total levels (Tomson *et al.*, 1994).

Schmidt and co-workers (1983) noted a correlation between noncompliance or sleep deprivation and a seizure relapse in 34 out of 50 pregnancies with increased seizure frequency. Further evidence for noncompliance as a major cause of seizure increase during pregnancy is given in the elaborate study by Otani (1985). He followed prospectively the course of 110 pregnancies of epileptic women and related the outcome to the patients' compliance with the prescribed drug therapy, as assessed through patient interviews and drug monitoring. Of the 25 subjects who showed an increase in seizure frequency, 52% were noncompliant with the drug therapy during pregnancy compared with 17% among the 85 pregnancies without deterioration in seizure control. Forty-three per cent of women noncompliant with drug therapy had an increase in seizures compared with 15% of those who took their drugs as prescribed. The author found that the most frequent reason for poor compliance during pregnancy was anxiety about the side-effects of antiepileptic drugs, including teratogenicity and possible harmful effects on the newborn by breast-feeding. This observation underlines the importance of pre-pregnancy counselling in the effort to optimize drug therapy during pregnancy. There is a pronounced variation in the percentage of women with epilepsy who have received counselling before pregnancy. For example, Wilhelm *et al.* (1990) reported pre-pregnancy counselling to occur in only 8.5% of cases compared with 43% in the prospective study from Stockholm (Tomson *et al.*, 1994). In the Stockholm study information on the topic was provided proactively and repeatedly to, among others, all maternity welfare units in the area.

CONCLUSIONS

Most studies of the effect of pregnancy on epilepsy have limitations that hamper the interpretation and complicate comparisons between the different studies. Nevertheless, previous retrospective and recent prospective data suggest that seizure control is unaffected by pregnancy in the majority of patients with epilepsy if the patients are managed during pregnancy according to the principles outlined in the study protocols. Labour and delivery appear to be the most sensitive periods in terms of seizure control, with a marked increase in seizure frequency compared with other periods of pregnancy. A deleterious effect of pregnancy on seizure control, outlasting pregnancy and puerperium appears to be rare. There is no consensus concerning epilepsy-related risk factors, but it is suggested that localization-related epilepsy and a high frequency of seizures before pregnancy may be associated with a higher risk of deterioration of seizure control during pregnancy. Poor compliance with the prescribed drug therapy is a major cause for seizure increase. This may in turn partly explain why failure to receive pre-pregnancy counselling has been identified as an important risk factor. As a consequence, efforts should be made to increase the number of patients who receive counselling before pregnancy in order to enhance seizure control.

REFERENCES

Bardy, A.H. (1987). Incidence of seizures during pregnancy, labour and puerperium in epileptic women: a prospective study. *Acta Neurol Scand* **75**, 356–360.
Canger, R., Avanzini, G., Battino, D. *et al.* (1982). Modifications of seizure frequency in pregnant patients with epilepsy: a prospective study. In: Janz, D., Dam, M., Richens, A., Bossi, L., Helge, H. and Schmidt, D. (Eds), *Epilepsy, Pregnancy, and the Child*. Raven Press, New York, pp. 33–38.
Cramer, J.A., Scheyer, R. and Mattson, R. (1990). Compliance declines between clinical visits. *Arch Intern Med* **150**, 1509–1510.
Dalessio, D.J. (1985). Seizure disorders and pregnancy. *N Engl J Med* **315**, 559–563.

Drislane, F.W. (1994). Persistent worsening of epilepsy associated with pregnancy. *J Epilepsy* **7**, 268–272.

Forsgren, L. (1992). Prevalence of epilepsy in adults in northern Sweden. *Epilepsia* **33**, 450–458.

Fröscher, W., Herrmann, R., Niesen, M., Bülau, P., Penin, H. and Hildenbrand, G. (1991). Untersuchungen zum Schwangerschaftsverlauf und zur Teratogenität der Antiepileptika bei 66 Epilepsie-Patientinnen. *Schweiz Arch Neurol Psychiatr* **142**, 389–407.

Gjerde, I.O., Strandjord, R.E. and Ulstein, M. (1988). The course of epilepsy during pregnancy: a study of 78 cases. *Acta Neurol Scand* **78**, 198–205.

Knight, A.H. and Rhind, E.G. (1975). Epilepsy and pregnancy: a study of 153 pregnancies in 59 patients. *Epilepsia* **16**, 99–110.

Lander, C.M. and Eadie, M.J. (1991). Plasma antiepileptic drug concentrations during pregnancy. *Epilepsia* **32**, 257–266.

Lopes-Cendes, I.E., Andermann, E., Cendes, L., Dansky, L. and Andermann, F. (1992). Risk factors for changes in seizure frequency during pregnancy of epileptic women: a cohort study. *Epilepsia* **33** (suppl 3), 57.

Nerlinger, H. (1889). Über die Epilepsie und das Fortpflanzungsgeschäft des Weibes in ihren gegenseitigen Beziehungen. Inaugural dissertation, Strassburg, Austria.

Otani, K. (1985). Risk factors for the increased seizure frequency during pregnancy and puerperium. *Folia Psychiatr Neurol Jap* **39**, 33–41.

Philbert, A. and Dam, M. (1982). The epileptic mother and her child. *Epilepsia* **23**, 85–99.

Remillard, G., Dansky, L., Andermann, E. and Andermann, F. (1982). Seizure frequency during pregnancy and the puerperium. In: Janz, D., Dam, M., Richens, A., Bossi, L., Helge, H. and Schmidt, D. (Eds), *Epilepsy, Pregnancy, and the Child*. Raven Press, New York, pp. 15–26.

Sabers, A. and Dam, M. (1990). Pregnancy, delivery and puerperium. In: Dam, M. and Gram, L. (Eds), *Comprehensive Epileptology*. Raven Press, New York, pp. 299–307.

Schmidt, D. (1982). The effect of pregnancy on the natural history of epilepsy: a review of the literature. In: Janz, D., Dam, M., Richens, A., Bossi, L., Helge, H. and Schmidt, D. (Eds), *Epilepsy, Pregnancy, and the Child*. Raven Press, New York, pp. 3–14.

Schmidt, D., Beck, B., Mannagetta, G., Janz, D. and Koch, S. (1982). The effect of pregnancy on the course of epilepsy: a prospective study. In: Janz, D., Dam, M., Richens, A., Bossi, L., Helge, H. and Schmidt, D. (Eds), *Epilepsy, Pregnancy, and the Child*. Raven Press, New York, pp. 39–49.

Schmidt, D., Canger, R., Avanzini, G. *et al.* (1983). Change of seizure frequency in pregnant epileptic women. *J Neurol Neurosurg Psychiatry* **46**, 751–755.

Tanganelli, P. and Regesta, G. (1992). Epilepsy, pregnancy, and major birth anomalies. *Neurology* **42** (suppl 5), 89–93.

Tomson, T., Lindbom, U., Ekqvist, B. and Sundqvist, A. (1994). Epilepsy and pregnancy: a prospective study of seizure control in relation to free and total plasma concentrations of carbamazepine and phenytoin. *Epilepsy* **35**, 122–130.

Wilhelm, J., Morris, D. and Hotham, N. (1990). Epilepsy and pregnancy: a review of 98 pregnancies. *Aust N Z J Obstet Gynaecol* **30**, 290–295.

12

Vitamin Supplementation

LENNART GRAM

Department of Neurology, State University Hospital, Copenhagen, Denmark

INTRODUCTION

Changes in the levels of vitamins, vitamin K and folates in the mother and fetus/child have been incriminated with regard to fetal abnormalities as well as complications in relation to labour and birth, in healthy volunteers as well as in women with epilepsy.

FOLATES

Women without epilepsy

In 1952, for the first time, an association was suggested between neural tube defects (NTD) and low folate levels, caused by the use of folate antagonists (Thiersch, 1952). This suspicion was later confirmed by Hibbard and Smithells (1965) who observed a link between folate deficiency and fetal malformations of the central nervous system, including NTD. It is well established that the frequency of NTD in spontaneous abortions is greatly increased (Byrne and Warburton, 1986) and it is interesting that by 1964 a possible relationship between spontaneous abortion and folate deficiency was demonstrated (Hibbard, 1964).

As a consequence, maternal shortage of folate during the periconceptional period may play a role in the development of NTD and therefore maternal folate supplementation in early pregnancy might be a preventive measure against the development of NTD.

To date five observational case–control studies have been performed, all of which recruited females without a previously NTD-affected pregnancy receiving folate supplementation of up to 0.8 mg/day (Bower and Stanley, 1989; Mulinare *et al.*, 1988; Milunsky *et al.*, 1989; Mills *et al.*, 1989; Werler *et al.*, 1993). All of these studies, except one (Mills *et al.*, 1989), showed significant risk reductions for giving birth to a child with NTD.

Table 1. Intervention studies of folate.

Authors, year	Investigation	Design	Study population	Supplementation: folate vs placebo	Result
Smithells et al., 1993	Nonrandomized, multicentre	Recurrence of NTD	973	0.36 mg folate + multivitamins	RR=0.14*
Vergel et al., 1990	Nonrandomized	Recurrence of NTD	195	5.0 mg folate	n.s.
Laurence et al., 1981	Randomized	Recurrence of NTD	111	4.0 mg folate	RR=0.40
MRC, 1991	Randomized, multicentre	Recurrence of NTD	1 195	4.0 mg folate	RR=0.28*
Czeizel and Dudás, 1992	Randomized	Occurrence of NTD	4 156	0.8 mg folate	s.r.

RR, relative risk; n.s., not significant; s.r., significant ($p = 0.029$) reduction in incidence of NTD.
*$p<0.05$.

A similar case–control study has been performed for orofacial clefts, demonstrating a significant risk reduction with folic acid supplementation of 0.4–0.8 mg/day for giving birth to a child with isolated cleft of palate and lip but not for multiple clefts of palate and lip, isolated and multiple cleft palates (Shaw et al., 1995).

In addition, a number of interventional studies have demonstrated the protective effect of periconceptional folate supplementation (Table 1). The majority of these comprised women with a history of previous NTD births supplemented with folates at least four weeks before conception and continuing throughout the first trimester.

Smithells and co-workers (1983), in a nonrandomized design, compared unsupplemented females with women receiving multivitamins and 0.36 mg/day of folates (total $n=1178$) and found a significant risk reduction of 86% of NTD.

In a similar design comprising 215 persons receiving 5.0 mg/day of folate, Vergel et al. (1990) observed a 100% risk reduction for the recurrence of NTD. However, due to the smaller number of persons participating the 95% confidence intervals (CI) are so wide as to render this result nonsignificant.

In a randomized design comprising 111 persons Laurence et al. (1981) investigated the protective effect of folic acid 4.0 mg/day and found a risk reduction of 58% which, considering the 95% CI, is not significant.

The largest randomized study investigating the effect of folate on the recurrence of NTD was undertaken by the Medical Research Council (MRC Vitamin Study Group, 1991). This recruited 1817 women of whom 1195 completed a pregnancy and thus could be analysed following either placebo, multivitamins without folic acid, 4.0 mg/day of folic acid, or folic acid plus multivitamins. Only folic acid showed a significant protection of 72% (95%

CI 0.12–0.71) for the recurrence of NTD. The other vitamins were without protective effect.

So far only one study has investigated the effect of folate supplementation on the first occurrence of NTD; this is important since the majority of NTD are single, sporadically occurring cases. Czeizel and Dudás (1992) randomized 7540 Hungarian women planning a pregnancy to supplementation either with multivitamins including 0.8 mg of folic acid or with trace elements including a low dose of vitamin C. Pregnancy was confirmed in 4753 women, of whom 48 were not traceable because of change of address or moving abroad. Thus pregnancy outcomes were evaluated in 99% of women becoming pregnant. A significant risk reduction in the incidence of neural tube defect was demonstrated, $p=0.029$.

Speculations about the mechanism by which decreased folic acid concentrations cause an increased frequency of NTD have emerged in the literature. Steegers-Theunissen et al. (1991) suggested that since folate is an important substrate in the metabolism of homocysteine, disturbance in the metabolism of this compound, folate deficiency giving rise to hyperhomocysteinaemia, could cause at least a subset of NTD. Methionine is required as the essential amino acid which is converted to homocysteine. Significant increased homocysteine levels have been demonstrated in women with unexplained recurrent early pregnancy loss, as well as in women giving birth to NTD children, compared with normal pregnancies (Wouters et al., 1993; Mills et al., 1995). In addition, a recent meta-analysis seems to suggest that hyperhomocysteinaemia may be a risk factor for the development of vascular disease (Boushey et al., 1995). Consequently, it is possible that there may be additional long-term benefits of folic acid supplementation in pregnant women.

Although folic acid is generally accepted as nontoxic in man, high doses (>1 mg/day) may mask the haematological effects of a vitamin B_{12} deficiency while the neurological manifestations progress (Herbert, 1992).

Women with epilepsy

It is well established that women taking antiepileptic drugs (AEDs) have an increased risk of giving birth to infants with congenital malformations, including NTDs (Kelly, 1984). Meadow (1968) had previously speculated that this could be due to a folate deficiency induced by AEDs. In particular, two AEDs have been associated with the occurrence of NTDs. For carbamazepine the risk is in the range of 0.5–1.0% (Rosa, 1991), while for valproate the risk is 1–2% (Lindhout and Schmidt, 1986).

A large number of studies have confirmed that non-pregnant women with epilepsy treated with AEDs have significantly lower folate levels in comparison with healthy controls. The mechanism responsible for this is probably the enzyme-inducing properties which the majority of the classical AEDs exhibit (Perucca, 1987). Consistent with this idea, no changes were found in serum or red blood cell folate concentrations following treatment with one of the novel, nonenzyme-inducing AEDs, lamotrigine (Sander and Patsalos, 1992). Despite the fact that valproate is not enzyme-inducing it seems to interfere with the metabolism of folate and thus predispose to the occurrence of NTDs (Wegner and Nau, 1992). A recent experimental study in rats and mice treated with valproate has demonstrated that administration of methionine significantly reduced the frequency of NTD offspring (Ehlers *et al.*, 1996), consistent with the previously mentioned apparent link between folate, cysteine and methionine.

In normal pregnancies folate levels progressively decline because of the increased folate requirements of the mother and fetus, suggesting that women with epilepsy taking enzyme-inducing AEDs may have an increased risk of developing a folate deficiency during their pregnancies. Consequently, Biale and Lewenthal (1984) undertook a study comparing persons with treated epilepsy, comprising historical controls, with women prospectively being supplemented with 2.5–5.0 mg folic acid per day. Although a significant reduction in the rate of malformations was claimed, due to the limited number of persons recruited the width of the 95% CI made the result nonsignificant.

Dansky *et al.* (1987) demonstrated that pregnant women with epilepsy had an increased frequency of folate deficiency which increased as the pregnancy progressed. In addition, a correlation was observed between low blood folate levels and pregnancies with an abnormal outcome. Females being supplemented with folic acid 0.1–5.0 mg/day (median 0.5 mg) achieved normal folate concentrations.

For women being treated with either valproate or carbamazepine, which apparently involve a risk for the first occurrence of a NTD (0.5–2.0%) in the same range as that for a recurrence of an NTD-pregnancy (3.5%) recommendations exist for supplementation with 4.0 mg/day of folic acid (Anonymous, 1994).

VITAMIN K

Women without epilepsy

Deficiency of vitamin K remains a significant worldwide cause of neonatal morbidity and mortality (Clarkson and James, 1990). The result may be three different patterns of bleeding in the neonatal period: early, within 24 hours of life; classic, occurring between the second to fifth days of life; and late haemorrhage, after the fifth day of life (Lane and Hathaway, 1985). Often the occurrence of an early haemorrhage is related to the use of medications during pregnancy that interfere with vitamin K synthesis in the fetus, among which are AEDs (Mountain *et al.*, 1970). Late haemorrhage, often involving major intracranial haemorrhage, is becoming increasingly recognized in breast-fed infants beyond one month of age who did not receive vitamin K prophylaxis after birth. As many as 50% of infants at the fifth day of life have a vitamin K deficiency (Shapiro *et al.*, 1986), and in premature neonates these abnormalities are even more prevalent. Apparently breast-fed neonates have an increased risk, compared with those fed products derived from cow's milk (Keenan *et al.*, 1971).

More recently, some controversy surrounds the route of administration of vitamin K prophylaxis in neonates, some investigators suggesting that oral administration be used instead of intramuscular injection (Brown *et al.*, 1989), while others oppose this view (Fetus and Newborn Committee, Canadian Pediatric Society, 1988). Oral prophylaxis has gained favour because of the suspicion that an association exists between parenteral vitamin K prophylaxis and the occurrence of leukaemia and other malignant conditions (Goldring *et al.*, 1992). This could not, however, be substantiated in subsequent case–control studies (Eklund *et al.*, 1993; Klebanoff *et al.*, 1993).

Women with epilepsy

The first report of an association between AED treatment and neonatal haemorrhage was in 1958 by van Crevald. The mechanism by which AEDs cause vitamin K deficiency involves their enzyme-inducing effect, combined with the fact that they readily cross the placenta and induce microsomal enzymes in the fetal liver (Cornelissen *et al.*, 1993a). Consistent with this the investigators did not find any adverse effect of valproate, which is not enzyme-inducing, on levels of vitamin K. The reason that AEDs provoke early bleeding in newborns, appearing within the first 24 hours of life, is that they are competitive inhibitors of prothrombin precursors. Results of mater-nal coagulation studies are often normal and this situation may not be prevented by perinatal vitamin K prophylaxis, but only by administering vitamin K to the mother during the last weeks of pregnancy, which has there-fore been recommended (Yerby, 1987).

Cornelissen *et al.* (1993b) undertook a case–control study supplementing mothers treated with enzyme-inducing AEDs with vitamin K 10 mg/day during the last month of their pregnancies. They found that this caused a normalization of vitamin K levels in cord blood of the neonates, and thus recommended antenatal vitamin K supplementation. Others have recom-mended combining antenatal supplementation and parenteral perinatal administration of vitamin K (Moslet and Hansen, 1991).

RECOMMENDATIONS

Folates

At national levels slightly different recommendations exist. In the UK a daily intake of 0.4 mg of folic acid is recommended (Report from an Expert Advisory Committee, 1992); identical recommendations exist in the USA (Center for Disease Control, 1993), in The Netherlands, Australia, New Zealand and China. In Norway current recommendations are that pregnant women should eat food rich in folates, whereby a daily intake of 0.3 mg is estimated, necessitating additional supplementation with 0.1 mg of folic acid in tablet form (Statens Helsetilsyn, 1993). However, these recommendations are currently being revised. In some countries, for example the USA, The Netherlands and Norway, recommendations are also given for women with a previous NTD pregnancy. In this situation supplementation with a daily dose of 4.0 mg of folic acid is advised. In Denmark recommendations are currently under consideration and are expected to be issued shortly.

In the previously published Consensus Guidelines it is recommended that all women with epilepsy undergoing treatment with AEDs receive daily folic acid (the amount is unspecified) in order to ensure that they maintain normal folic acid concentrations in serum and red blood cells during the first trimester (Delgado-Escueta and Janz, 1992).

The recommendations published in this volume suggest daily supplementation with 0.4 mg of folic acid. In case of a previous NTD pregnancy a dose of 4.0 mg of folic acid is recommended. Since documentation of efficacy is lacking the question of whether persons treated with enzyme-inducing AEDs should also receive 4.0 mg/day of folic acid is left open.

Vitamin K

The Consensus Guidelines recommend antenatal vitamin K supplementation 20 mg/day for the last month of pregnancy, combined with 1 mg of parenteral vitamin K administered to the newborn (Delagado-Escueta and Janz, 1992).

Recommendations published in this volume (Chapter 20) are more cautious, stating that some recommend antenatal supplementation with 10 mg/day of vitamin K for the last month of pregnancy in women treated with enzyme-inducing AEDs. General agreement exists that parenteral administration of 1 mg of vitamin K immediately after birth should be given, while different opinions exist with regard to continuing peroral treatment with vitamin K of the infant for the first three months of life. The Danish National Health Board currently recommends that breast-fed infants receive 1 mg/week of vitamin K given perorally for the first three months of life, while antenatal vitamin K supplementation is not recommended.

REFERENCES

Anonymous (1994). Epilepsy and pregnancy. *Drug Ther Bull* **32**, 49–51.

Biale, Y. and Lewenthal, H. (1984). Effect of folic acid supplementation on congenital malformations due to anticonvulsant drugs. *Eur J Gynaecol Reprod Biol* **18**, 211–216.

Boushey, C.J., Bereford, S.A.A., Omenn, G.S. and Motulsky, A.G. (1995). A quantitative assessment of plasma homocysteine as a risk factor for vascular disease. *JAMA* **274**, 1049–1057.

Bower, C., Stanley, F.J. (1989). Dietary folate as a risk factor for neural tube defects: evidence from a case control study in Western Australia. *Med J Aust* **150**, 613–619.

Brown, S.G., McHugh, G. and Shapeleski, J. (1989). Should intramuscular vitamin K prophylaxis for hemorragic disease of the newborn be continued? A decision analysis. *N Z J Med* **102**, 3–5.

Byrne, J. and Warburton, D. (1986). Neural tube defects in spontaneous abortions. *Am J Med Genet* **25**, 327–333.

Center for Disease Control (1993). Recommendations for the use of folic acid to reduce the number of neuronal tube defects. *JAMA* **269**, 1233–1238.

Clarkson, P.M. and James, A.G. (1990). Parenteral vitamin K_1: the effective prophylaxis against hemorrhagic disease for all newborn infants. *N Z Med J* **103**, 95–96.

Cornelissen, M., Steegers-Theunissen, R., Kollée, L., Eskes, T., Motohara, K. and Monnens, L. (1993a). Supplementation of vitamin K in pregnant women receiving anticonvulsant therapy prevents neonatal vitamin K deficiency. *Am J Obstet Gynecol* **168**, 884–888.

Cornelissen, M., Steegers-Theunissen, R., Kollée, L. *et al.* (1993b). Increased incidence of neonatal vitamin K deficiency resulting from maternal anticonvulsant therapy. *Am J Obstet Gynecol* **168**, 923–928.

Czeizel, A.E. and Dudás, I. (1992). Prevention of the first occurrence of neural tube defects by periconceptional vitamin supplementation. *N Engl J Med* **327**, 1832–1835.

Dansky, L.W., Andermann, E., Rosenblatt, D. *et al.* (1987). Anticonvulsants, folate levels, and pregnancy outcome: a prospective study. *Ann Neurol* **21**, 176–182.

Delgado-Escueta, A.V. and Janz, D. (1992). Consensus guidelines: preconception counselling, management and care of the pregnant woman with epilepsy. *Neurology* **42** (suppl 5), 149–160.

Ehlers, K., Elmazar, M.M.A. and Nau, H. (1996). Methionine reduces the valproic acid-induced spina bifida rate in mice without altering valproic acid kinetics. *J Nutr* **126**, 67–75.

Eklund, H., Finnström, O. and Gunnarskov, J. (1993). Administration of vitamin K to newborn infants and childhood cancer. *BMJ* **307**, 89–91.

Fetus and Newborn Committee, Canadian Pediatric Society (1988). The use of vitamin K in the perinatal period. *Can Med Assoc J* **139**, 127–130.

Goldring, J., Greenwood, R., Birmingham, K. and Mott, M. (1992). Childhood cancer, intramuscular vitamin K and pethidine given during labour. *BMJ* **305**, 341–346.

Herbert, V. (1992). Folate and neural tube defects. *Nutr Today* November, 30–33.

Hibbard, B.M. (1964). The role of folic acid in pregnancy. With particular references to anaemia, abruption and abortion. *Gynaecol Br Commonw* **71**, 529–542.

Hibbard, E.D. and Smithells, R.W. (1965). Folic acid metabolism and human embryopathy (Letter). *Lancet* **i**, 1254.

Kelly, T.E. (1984). Teratogenicity of anticonvulsant drugs I: review of the literature. *Am J Med Genet* **19**, 413–458.

Keenan, W.J., Jewett, T. and Glueck, H.I. (1971). Role of feeding and vitamin K in hypothrombinaemia of the newborn. *Am J Dis Child* **121**, 127–137.

Klebanoff, M.A., Read, J.S. and Mills, J.L. (1993). The risk of childhood cancer after neonatal exposure to vitamin K. *N Engl J Med* **329**, 905–908.

Lane, P.A. and Hathaway, W.E. (1985). Vitamin K in infancy. *J Pediatr* **106**, 351–359.

Laurence, K.M., James, J., Miller, M.H., Tennant, G.B. and Campbell, H. (1981). Double-blind randomised controlled trial of folate treatment before conception to prevent recurrence of neural-tube defects. *BMJ* **282**, 1509–1511.

Lindhout, D. and Schmidt, D. (1986). *In-utero* exposure to valproate and neural tube defects. *Lancet* **ii**, 1392–1393.

Meadow, S.R. (1968). Anticonvulsant drugs and congenital abnormalities. *Lancet* **ii**, 1296.

Mills, J.L., Rhoads, G.G. and Simpson, J.L. (1989). The absence of a relation between the periconceptional use of vitamins and neural tube defects. *N Engl J Med* **321**, 430–435.

Mills, J.L., McPartlin, J.M., Kirke, P.N., Lee, Y.J., Conley, M.R. and Weir, D.G. (1995). Homocysteine metabolism in pregnancies complicated by neural-tube defects. *Lancet* **345**, 791.

Milunsky, A., Jick, H. and Jick, S.S. (1989). Multivitamin/folic acid supplementation in early pregnancy reduces the prevalence of neural tube defects. *JAMA* **262**, 2847–2852.

Moslet, U. and Hansen, E.S. (1991). A review of vitamin K, epilepsy and pregnancy. *Acta Neurol Scand* **85**, 39–43.

Mountain, K.R., Hirsch, J. and Gallus, A.S. (1970). Neonatal coagulation defects due to anticonvulsant drug treatment in pregnancy. *Lancet* **i**, 265–268.

MRC Vitamin Study Group (1991). Prevention of neural tube defects: results of the Medical Research Council Vitamin Study. *Lancet* **338**, 131–137.

Mulinare, J., Cordero, F.J., Erickson, J.D. and Berry, R.J. (1988). Periconceptional use of multivitamins and the occurrence of neural tube defects. *JAMA* **260**, 3141–3145.

Perucca, E. (1987). Clinical implications of hepatic microsomal enzyme induction by antiepileptic drugs. *Pharmacol Ther* **33**, 139–144.

Report from an Expert Advisory Committee (1992). *Folic Acid and the Prevention of Neural Tube Defects*. Department of Health, London, 1992.

Rosa, F.W. (1991). Spina bifida in infants of women treated with carbamazepine during pregnancy. *N Engl J Med* **324**, 674–677.

Sander, J.W.A.S. and Patsalos, P.N. (1992). An assessment of serum and red cell folate concentrations in patients with epilepsy on lamotrigine therapy. *Epilepsy Res* **13**, 89–92.

Shapiro, A.D., Jacobsen, L.J. and Armon, M.E. (1986). Vitamin K deficiency in the newborn infant: prevalence and perinatal risk factors. *J Pediatr* **106**, 675–680.

Shaw, G.M. Lammer, E.J., Wasserman, C.R., O'Malley, C.D. and Tolarova, M.M. (1995). Risk of orofacial clefts in children born to women using multivitamins containing folic acid periconceptionally. *Lancet* **345**, 393–396.

Smithells, R.W., Nevin, N.C., Seller, M.J. *et al.* (1993). Further experience of vitamin supplementation for prevention of neural tube defect recurrences. *Lancet* **i**, 1027–1031.

Statens Helsetilsyn (1993). Tiltak som kan redusere forekomst av nevralrorsdefekter. *Rundskriv* **IK-4**, 93.

Steegers-Theunissen, R.P.M., Boers, G.H.J., Tijbels, J.M.F. and Eskes, T.K.A.B. (1991). Neural-tube defects and derangement of homocysteine metabolism. *N Engl J Med* **324**, 199–200.

Thiersch, J.B. (1952). Therapeutic abortions with a folic acid antagonist 4-amino-pteroylglutamic acid administration. *J Pediatr* **70**, 670–686.

van Crevald, S. (1958). Nouveaux aspects de la maladie hemorragique du nouveau-né. *Arch Fr Pediatr* **15**, 721–735.

Vergel, R.G., Sanchez, L.R., Heredero, B.L., Rodriguez, P.L. and Martinez, A.J. (1990). Primary prevention of neural tube defects with folic acid supplementation: Cuban experience. *Prenat Diagn* **10**, 149–152.

Wegner, C.H. and Nau, H. (1992). Alterations of embryonic folate metabolism by valproic acid during organogenesis: implications for the mechanism of teratogenesis. *Neurology* **42**, 17–24.

Werler, M.M., Shapiro, S. and Michell, A.A. (1993). Periconceptional folic acid exposure and risk of occurrent neural tube defects. *JAMA* **269**, 1257–1261.

Wouters, G.A.J., Boers, G.H.J., Blom, H.J. *et al.* (1993). Hyperhomocysteinemia: a risk factor in women with unexplained recurrent early pregnancy loss. *Fertil Steril* **60**, 820–825.

Yerby, M. (1987). Problems and management of the pregnant woman with epilepsy. *Epilepsia* **28** (suppl 3), 29–36.

Epilepsy and Pregnancy
Edited by T. Tomson, L. Gram, M. Sillanpää and S.I. Johannessen
© 1997 Wrightson Biomedical Publishing Ltd

13

Effects of Maternal Seizures on the Fetus

VILHO HIILESMAA
Departments of Obstetrics and Gynaecology, Helsinki University, Helsinki, Finland

INTRODUCTION

About 0.5–1.0% of pregnant women have epilepsy. Most of them are already on antiepileptic medication when pregnancy ensues. In spite of the general efficacy of modern antiepileptic drugs, occurrence of seizures during pregnancy cannot be completely avoided. In order to provide their young female patients with appropriate counselling before and during pregnancy, neurologists and obstetricians should be aware of the possible effects of maternal seizures on the fetus. In this chapter, the literature pertinent to the short-term and long-term fetal effects of maternal seizures during pregnancy and labour is reviewed.

LACTIC ACIDOSIS AFTER GENERALIZED TONIC-CLONIC SEIZURES

Profound alterations in acid-base equilibrium occur immediately after a generalized tonic-clonic seizure. This was demonstrated by Orringer *et al.* (1977) who took consecutive blood samples from eight patients immediately after a single generalized tonic-clonic seizure (GTCS). At 0–4 minutes after the seizure, the patients had a metabolic acidosis with a mean arterial pH of 7.14 (range 6.86–7.36). This acidosis was attributable, in large part, to the accumulation of lactate. Lactate levels ranged from 8.9 to 16.0, with a mean of 12.7 meq/l (normal values 0.3–1.5). Within one hour after the seizure the initially low pH had returned to normal whereas the lactate levels were still markedly elevated at a mean of 6.6 meq/l.

The metabolic changes in a pregnant woman after a GTCS are most probably transferred to her fetus. Although direct evidence of this in the form of blood analyses is missing, registrations of fetal heart rate during and immediately after a maternal GTCS in labour are compatible with fetal acidosis (Teramo *et al.*, 1979; Grunert and Field, 1985; Hiilesmaa *et al.*, 1985; Yerby, 1987). Typical reasons for fetal acidosis (much more common than maternal seizures) include placental insufficiency and umbilical cord compression. Low pH values at birth are associated with an increased risk of neonatal morbidity. There is thus a good reason to avoid situations which produce pronounced acidosis during pregnancy and labour, including maternal GTCS.

OTHER POSSIBLE EFFECTS OF MATERNAL GENERALIZED TONIC-CLONIC SEIZURES

In addition to lactic acidosis, a GTCS can have other effects. In animal experiments it causes marked, acute cardiovascular changes and an associated redistribution of the circulation. Blood pressure is elevated, blood flow increased in the common carotid artery and reduced in certain visceral arteries (Doba *et al.*, 1975). There are no animal experiments on uterine and placental blood flow during maternal seizures. Whether uterine blood flow decreases and contributes to the development of fetal acidosis during a maternal seizure in humans is not known.

It has been speculated that mechanical pressure on the uterus caused by convulsive contractions of the maternal abdominal muscles could reduce the uterine blood flow, and that certain humoral factors with effects upon the uteroplacental circulation could be excreted during a seizure. However, there is no proof of the existence of these mechanisms. A large uterus is susceptible to a contusion trauma if the patient falls during an unexpected GTCS.

The case-report by Goetting and Davidson (1987) suggests that fetal bradycardia during maternal seizures is due to hypoxia and acidosis, not to other factors.

EFFECTS OF SEIZURE TYPES OTHER THAN GENERALIZED TONIC-CLONIC SEIZURES

It is obvious that partial seizures and nonconvulsive generalized seizures do not produce the same pronounced metabolic effects as those that follow a GTCS. It is thus unlikely that these seizure types pose similar immediate risks to the fetus. However, partial seizures can be very disturbing to the patient, more so when she is pregnant.

MATERNAL SEIZURES AND FETAL MALFORMATIONS

The prospective studies on epilepsy and pregnancy do not provide evidence of an association between maternal generalized convulsions during pregnancy and malformations (Gaily *et al.*, 1988a; Oguni *et al.*, 1992; Steegers-Theunissen *et al.*, 1994). The retrospective studies are unreliable in this respect due to poor information on the occurrence of seizures.

The thus far negative findings as to the teratogenicity of maternal seizures should not be taken as proof of their safety to the fetus. Organogenesis is a very short period of time, and few patients experience seizures during that time. Thus, very large controlled prospective studies would be needed to properly assess (or exclude) the teratogenic potential of seizures in humans. There are isolated reports indicating that a severe hypoxia in the mother can be teratogenic (Goodlin *et al.*, 1984).

SEIZURES AND OBSTETRIC COMPLICATIONS

An excess of almost all of the common pregnancy complications has been reported in women with epilepsy. These include toxaemia, preeclampsia, abortion, bleeding in pregnancy, placental abruption, and premature labour (Yerby *et al.*, 1985; Sonneveld and Correy, 1990; Wilhelm *et al.*, 1990; Steegers-Theunissen *et al.*, 1994). Although the metabolic, circulatory, and mechanical effects of maternal generalized tonic-clonic seizures could theoretically explain some of these obstetric complications, such as abortion, bleeding, placental abruption and premature labour, no such direct association has been verified. This does not exclude the possibility of such an association since seizure histories may be missing or are poorly recorded in retrospective and register-based studies.

In the prospective study of Steegers-Theunissen *et al.* (1994) no association was found between the seizures and abnormal pregnancy outcome. Some of the obstetric series show minimal or no increase in pregnancy complications among women with epilepsy (Egenaes, 1982; Hiilesmaa *et al.*, 1985). Although a healthy fetus seems to be remarkably resistant to a maternal seizure, hazardous situations can develop when a seizure occurs in a patient who already has a pre-existing obstetric problem.

Virtually all published reports agree that there is a 1.2–3 times increase in perinatal mortality, i.e. stillbirths and deaths of the neonate during the first week of life (Fedrick, 1973; Nelson and Ellenberg, 1982; Egenaes, 1982; Hiilesmaa *et al.*, 1985). Intrauterine deaths immediately after a seizure have been reported only occasionally (Higgins and Comerford, 1974).

It can be assumed that the intrauterine death of a healthy fetus after a maternal GTCS must be very rare, since many women have such seizures during pregnancy in spite of antiepileptic medication. For example, Bardy (1982) reported on a total of 152 GTCS during pregnancy in 154 women with epilepsy. None of the seizures was followed by immediate fetal death or obstetric complication. We must, therefore, look for explanations other than seizures for the consistently reported increase in perinatal mortality in women with epilepsy. Perhaps the aetiology is multifactorial (Hiilesmaa, 1992).

STATUS EPILEPTICUS DURING PREGNANCY

The reports published decades ago on status epilepticus during pregnancy showed a high maternal and fetal mortality. Immediate interruption of the pregnancy was commonly considered a necessary part of the treatment. Teramo and Hiilesmaa (1982) compiled 29 cases from medical literature. Nine of the mothers died, and at least 14 of the fetuses died *in utero* or shortly after birth.

The advances in antiepileptic treatment and in the care of premature and asphyxiated babies since the 1960s have vastly improved the chances of survival for the mother and the fetus after a status epilepticus during pregnancy. Several recent case-reports and small series indicate that status epilepticus can be halted with drugs and the pregnancy continued (Ramsay *et al.*, 1978; Grunert and Field, 1985; Fougner *et al.*, 1985; Bag *et al.*, 1989; Méndez-Quijada *et al.*, 1990).

Although the therapeutic effect of delivery (usually by caesarean section) on a status epilepticus has not been well established, it should be considered for both fetal and maternal reasons (Grunert and Field, 1985; Thomas *et al.*, 1991). After 36 weeks of pregnancy, problems associated with prematurity are minimal. Provided expert care is available premature infants born at 28–32 weeks also have an excellent prognosis.

SEIZURES DURING LABOUR

GTCS during labour cause transient fetal asphyxia, as evidenced by cardiotocographic monitoring. Fetal bradycardia, reduced variability, and decelerations are seen for about 30 minutes after a seizure (Teramo *et al.*, 1979; Hiilesmaa *et al.*, 1985; Yerby, 1987). A prompt caesarean section should then be considered, to lessen fetal risks and because of the reduced postictal ability of the mother to co-operate further.

A GTCS occurs during labour in about 1–2% of women with epilepsy and within 24 hours of delivery in another 1–2% (Bardy, 1982). Although these absolute figures are small, the probability of a seizure during labour and during the first postpartum day is nine times greater than the average probability of a seizure during pregnancy (Bardy, 1982).

Goetting and Davidson (1987) reported on a patient in labour who had a 70-minute tonic-clonic convulsion. Maternal acid-base status and oxygenation remained normal. Fetal monitoring showed no evidence of distress. This case suggests that fetal bradycardia during maternal seizures is not developed unless the mother develops acidosis.

MATERNAL SEIZURES AND THE CHILD'S PSYCHOMOTOR AND INTELLECTUAL DEVELOPMENT

The risk of psychomotor retardation and the prevalence of mental subnormality are slightly increased in offspring of mothers with epilepsy (Granström and Gaily, 1992). This probably reflects the synergistic effects of many factors connected with maternal epilepsy. Of these, exposure to drugs has been the most intensively studied. The impact of other factors such as seizures during pregnancy, type and duration of maternal epilepsy, inherited brain disorders, and nonoptimal psychosocial environment, remain much less studied and less well understood. In most studies it has been difficult specifically to address the effects of seizures on the child's development (Granström and Gaily, 1992).

Prolonged severe hypoxia in the mother could have a catastrophic effect on the child's brain (Goodlin et al., 1984). Isolated brief seizures, although generalized, obviously do not have the same harmful fetal effect as prolonged seizures, since no association has been found between the occurrence of maternal generalized convulsions and psychomotor retardation of the child in the prospective studies focusing on the subject (Fujioka et al., 1984; Gaily et al., 1988b).

Gaily et al. (1990) reported that the occurrence of GTCS during pregnancy was associated with an increased risk for specific cognitive dysfunction in the offspring. The authors found that the risk of cognitive deficits was also high in children exposed only to nonconvulsive maternal seizures. It thus seems unlikely that fetal asphyxia due to seizures could be the only explanation. The authors suggest that this association also reflects the heredity of the other central nervous system findings connected with the epilepsy of the mother.

REFERENCES

Bag, S., Behari, M., Ahuja, G.K. and Karmakar, M.G. (1989). Pregnancy and epilepsy. *J Neurol* **5**, 311–313.

Bardy, A. (1982). Epilepsy and pregnancy. A prospective study of 154 pregnancies in epileptic women [Thesis]. University of Helsinki, Finland.

Doba, N., Beresford, H.R. and Reis, D.J. (1975). Changes in regional blood flow and cardiodynamics with electrically and chemically induced epilepsy in cat. *Brain Res* **90**, 115–132.

Egenaes, J. (1982). Outcome of pregnancy in women with epilepsy, Norway 1967–1978: complications during pregnancy and delivery. In: Janz, D., Dam, M., Richens, A., Bossi, L., Helge, H. and Schmidt, D. (Eds), *Epilepsy, Pregnancy, and the Child*. Raven Press, New York, pp. 81–85.

Fedrick, J. (1973). Epilepsy and pregnancy: a report from the Oxford Record Linkage Study. *BMJ* **2**, 442–448.

Fougner, A.C., Wilson, S.J. and Selzer, V.L. (1985). Status epilepticus in pregnancy. A case report. *J Reprod Med* **30**, 948–950.

Fujioka, K., Kaneko, S., Hirano, T., Fujita, S., Sato, T. and Matsui, M. (1984). In: Sato, T. and Shinagawa, S. (Eds), *Antiepileptic Drugs and Pregnancy*. Excerpta Medica, Amsterdam, pp. 196–206.

Gaily, E., Granström, M.-L., Hiilesmaa, V. and Bardy, A. (1988a). Minor anomalies in offspring of epileptic mothers. *J Pediatr* **112**, 520–529.

Gaily, E., Kantola-Sorsa, E. and Granström, M.-L. (1988b). Intelligence of children of epileptic mothers. *J Pediatr* **113**, 677–684.

Gaily, E., Kantola-Sorsa, E. and Granström, M.-L. (1990). Specific cognitive dysfunction in children with epileptic mothers. *Dev Med Child Neurol* **32**, 403–414.

Goetting, M.G. and Davidson, B.N. (1987). Status epilepticus during labor. A case report. *J Reprod Med* **32**, 313–314.

Goodlin, R.C., Heidrick, W.P., Papenfuss, H.L. and Kubitz, R.L. (1984). Fetal malformations associated with maternal hypoxia. *Am J Obstet Gynecol* **149**, 228–229.

Granström, M.-L. and Gaily, E. (1992). Psychomotor development in children of mothers with epilepsy. *Neurology* **42** (suppl 5), 144–148.

Grunert, G.M. and Field, D.R. (1985). Refractory status epilepticus in pregnancy. A case report. *J Reprod Med* **30**, 69–73.

Higgins, T.A. and Comerford, J.B. (1974). Epilepsy in pregnancy. *J Ir Med Assoc* **67**, 317–320.

Hiilesmaa, V.K. (1992). Pregnancy and birth in women with epilepsy. *Neurology* **42** (suppl 5), 8–11.

Hiilesmaa, V.K., Bardy, A.H. and Teramo, K. (1985). Obstetric outcome in women with epilepsy. *Am J Obstet Gynecol* **152**, 499–504.

Méndez-Quijada, J., Mores, A.F. and Juvinao, N. (1990). Status epilepticus in pregnancy. A case report. *J Reprod Med* **35**, 289–291.

Nelson, K.B. and Ellenberg, J.H. (1982). Maternal seizure disorder, outcome of pregnancy, and neurologic abnormalities in the children. *Neurology* **32**, 1247–1254.

Oguni, M., Dansky, L., Andermann, E., Sherwin, A. and Andermann, F. (1992). Improved pregnancy outcome in epileptic women in the last decade: relationship to maternal anticonvulsant therapy. *Brain Res* **14**, 371–380.

Orringer, C.E., Eustace, J.C., Wunsch, C.D. and Gardner, L.B. (1977). Natural history of lactic acidosis after grand-mal seizures. A model for the study of an anion-gap acidosis not associated with hyperkalemia. *N Engl J Med* **297**, 796–799.

Ramsay, R.E., Strauss, R.G., Wilder, B.J. and Willmore, L.J. (1978). Status epilepticus in pregnancy: effect of phenytoin malasborbtion on seizure control. *Neurology* **28**, 85–89.

Sonneveld, S.W. and Correy, J.F. (1990). Outcome of pregnancies complicated by epilepsy in Tasmania, 1981–1988. *Aust N Z J Obstet Gynaecol* **30**, 286–289.

Steegers-Theunissen, R.P.M., Renier, W.O., Borm, G.F. *et al.* (1994). Factors influencing the risk of abnormal pregnancy outcome in epileptic women: a multicentre prospective study. *Epilepsy Res* **18**, 261–269.

Teramo, K., Hiilesmaa, V., Bardy, A. and Saarikoski, S. (1979). Fetal heart rate during a maternal grand mal epileptic seizure. *J Perinat Med* **7**, 3–6.

Teramo, K. and Hiilesmaa, V.K. (1982). Pregnancy and fetal complications in epileptic pregnancies. In: Janz, D., Dam, M., Richens, A., Bossi, L., Helge, H. and Schmidt, D. (Eds), *Epilepsy, Pregnancy and the Child*. Raven Press, New York, pp. 53–59.

Thomas, P., Barres, P. and Chatel, M. (1991). Complex partial status epilepticus of extratemporal origin: report of case. *Neurology* **41**, 1147–1149.

Wilhelm, J., Morrid, D. and Hotham, N. (1990). Epilepsy and pregnancy: a review of 98 pregnancies. *Aust N Z J Obstet Gynaecol* **30**, 290–295.

Yerby, M.S. (1987). Problems and management of the pregnant woman with epilepsy. *Epilepsia* **28** (suppl 3), 29–36.

Yerby, M., Koepsell, T. and Daling, J. (1985). Pregnancy complications and outcomes in a cohort of women with epilepsy. *Epilepsia* **26**, 631–635.

Epilepsy and Pregnancy
Edited by T. Tomson, L. Gram, M. Sillanpää and S.I. Johannessen
© 1997 Wrightson Biomedical Publishing Ltd

14

Prenatal Diagnosis of Malformations

WIGGO FISCHER-RASMUSSEN
*Department of Obstetrics and Gynaecology, Hvidovre Hospital,
University of Copenhagen, Hvidovre, Denmark*

INTRODUCTION

The teratogenic impact of the major antiepileptic drugs, carbamazepine and valproate, together with the older phenytoin and phenobarbital, is debated elsewhere. It is not known which is the most teratogenic or causes more malformations. Neither is it known for sure whether the antiepileptic drugs induce specific malformation syndromes; however, neural tube defects have been especially associated with valproate and carbamazepine (Lindhout *et al*., 1984; Lindhout and Schmidt, 1986; Vestermark, 1993).

As the incidence of fetal malformations is increased in women with epilepsy approximately twofold (3%), and especially in those undergoing polytherapy (10%) (Lindhout *et al*., 1984), pregnant women with epilepsy should be considered high-risk patients and be offered prenatal examination for major fetal malformations.

Amniocentesis and ultrasound examination are capable of detecting neural tube defects, cardiac anomalies, and a range of deformities. There is no evidence of an increased frequency of chromosomal aberrations among the offspring of mothers with epilepsy. Ultrasound imaging plays a dominant role in antenatal diagnosis. The following is a brief exposé of the possibilities which can be offered by an obstetric department with a 'level 2' centre for ultrasound examination. For details and advanced diagnostic procedures the specific literature should be consulted.

PREGNANCY AND EPILEPSY: PRECONCEPTIONAL COUNSELLING AND SURVEILLANCE

The need for guidelines for women with epilepsy and pregnancy has been met in the USA (Delgado-Escueta and Janz, 1992). The guidelines include information for the woman who is planning pregnancy regarding monitoring

Table 1. Congenital malformations and fetal distress: precautions and interventions with respect to women with epilepsy.

Gestational age	Mother: precautions/interventions	Fetus: preventive and diagnostic aspects
Prior to pregnancy	Monotherapy Seizure control Vitamin supplementation Lifestyle	Reducing number of malformations

First trimester, early second trimester	Amniocentesis:
	   amnion alpha-fetoprotein
	   chromosome analysis
	Ultrasound examination
		Detecting malformations
		Dating of gestational age

Second and third trimesters	Surveillance:
	   seizures
	   drug compliance
	   blood concentration of drug
	   obstetrical complications
	   cardiotocography
	   ultrasound
	
	Vitamin K
		Prevention of fetal asphyxia
		
		Signs of:
		   asphyxia
		   intrauterine growth
		      retardation
		Prevention of intracranial haemorrhages

Delivery	Cardiotocography Tonic-clonic seizure control	Perinatal asphyxia Vitamin K
Postnatal period	Reduction of drug dosage	Excitation Sedation Suckling

during pregnancy, delivery and the postnatal period. Guidelines must be achieved in a consensus between the specialties of neurology, genetics, obstetrics and paediatrics. The information has to be disseminated into general practice but any fertile woman with epilepsy should – when her diagnosis of epilepsy is established – be informed that certain precautions should be taken prior to pregnancy and in early pregnancy. This could be the duty of the neurologist making the diagnosis but, as epilepsy usually is a disease of many years' duration the closest medical adviser to the woman at the time she is considering conception may often be her general practitioner. Once pregnancy has been achieved close co-operation between general practitioner, obstetrician and neurologist is important (Table 1).

A woman with epilepsy must be informed about fetal malformations when the issue of planning a pregnancy is brought up by her. To our present knowledge it is probable that epilepsy (depending on type) carries a genetic predisposition for birth defects and it is also probable that this risk may be further increased by antiepileptic drugs. Monotherapy is preferable to polytherapy and the influence on birth defects is greater for some antiepileptic drugs than for others.

At the preconceptional counselling stage the woman must be informed of the possibilities of antenatal diagnosis and its consequences. The antenatal diagnosis of a malformation may indicate referral of the pregnant woman to a centre where appropriate surgery can be carried out on the newborn. However, it may also imply a decision to induce abortion, depending on ethics, religion and legislation.

In preconceptional counselling it is justifiable to emphasize that the majority of pregnancies in women with epilepsy are uncomplicated provided there is good antenatal care and good seizure control with the lowest possible plasma level of the antiepileptic drug that protects against tonic-clonic convulsions. Frequent obstetrical checks would appear to be advisable as a slight increase in some common complications of pregnancy such as preeclampsia, haemorrhage, preterm labour and intrauterine growth retardation have been reported for women with epilepsy, but there is no agreement on this. Some studies report a threefold increase while others fail to demonstrate any difference from the general population. However, frequent antenatal visits may be of psychological importance to the pregnant woman with epilepsy. The obstetrician is able to reassure her that most women with epilepsy will have an uneventful vaginal delivery without convulsions, which is a common fear. She can be reassured of delivery by the vaginal route and that a caesarean section will only be performed if there are obstetrical indications, and not because of the epilepsy. Furthermore, she needs reassurance of the possibility of breast-feeding her baby despite the antiepileptic drug intake.

BIRTH DEFECTS

Major congenital malformations

Major malformations of serious significance to the infant are structural defects induced in early embryonic life during the development of an organ system. Types of major malformations are cleft lip/palate, cardiac diseases, cardiovascular malformations, intestinal atresia, urogenital deformities and neural tube defects. It is claimed that the pattern of malformations has changed following the institution of monotherapy (Lindhout et al., 1984; Källén, 1986; Kaneko et al., 1988), neural tube defects and hypospadias being the most frequent at present.

Birth defects such as meningomyelocele, cleft lip and ventricular septal defect indicate teratogenic effects in the very early embryonic period within 28 to 42 days after the first day of the last menstrual period. Often the woman will not yet have recognized her pregnant state.

Minor congenital malformations

Whereas the major malformations may disable the infant or demand surgical intervention, the minor malformations are structural defects which do not severely damage the individual. Types of minor malformations reported associated with antiepileptic drugs are: unusual morphologic facial features (hypertelorism, epicanthal folds, nasal deformities, low, rotated ears, long philtrum), digital hypoplasia, club foot, equino-varus and hypospadias.

PRENATAL DIAGNOSTIC METHODS (TABLE 2)

Maternal serum alpha-fetoprotein

For many years, it has been known that a very high concentration of alpha-fetoprotein (AFP) in the amniotic fluid and to a lesser degree in maternal serum occurs in mothers with fetuses suffering from neural tube defects (e.g. Kjessler and Johansson, 1977). Elevated concentrations of AFP may also be measured in cases of abdominal wall defects and certain renal diseases (e.g. congenital nephrosis of Finnish type). Screening for fetal malformations by maternal serum AFP at week 18 has in some studies (Nørgaard-Pedersen *et al.*, 1985) proven to be able to detect almost all cases of anencephaly, 80% of the spina bifidas, and 75% of the abdominal wall defects in a population with low incidence of neural tube defects (1 : 1 000 births). The condition for using AFP is a reliable determination of the gestational age. In many pregnant woman (15–25%) a safe gestational age can only be obtained by ultrasound measurement of the biparietal diameter at week 16–18 due to irregular periods or uncertain dating of the first day of the last menstrual period.

The frequent occurrence of elevated serum AFP concentration in the first drawn blood sample leads to a second sample. If the AFP concentration is

Table 2. Methods in the prenatal diagnosis of malformations.

Methods	Gestational age at application (completed week)	Principal diagnostic aim
Maternal serum alpha-fetoprotein (AFP)	16	Neural tube defects Down's syndrome
Chorionic villus sampling	8–10	Chromosomal disorders
Amniocentesis	15–16	Chromosomal disorders Neural tube defects (AFP)
Ultrasound	18–20	Malformations of organs: central nervous system cardiovascular system skeletal system and oral clefts urinary system gastrointestinal system

still elevated ultrasound examination and amniocentesis will be offered. The time required for this elucidation can easily run to more than a week leaving the pregnant woman with uncertainty regarding fetal well-being and outcome. This negatively emotional event at a time of psychic vulnerability causes many women to decline the test (Jørgensen, 1995).

Low serum levels of AFP occur in mothers having fetuses with Down's syndrome. As an alternative to the invasive procedures of chorionic villus sampling or amniocentesis, pregnant women in some countries are offered screening for Down's syndrome (or malformations) by serum determination of AFP in combination with human chorionic gonadotropin and unconjugated oestriol. The principal problems of screening of the pregnant population with regard to methods and indications have recently been elucidated by the British Royal College of Obstetricians and Gynaecologists (RCOG, 1993). It must be emphasized that determination of maternal serum AFP is a screening procedure and not a diagnostic tool.

Chorionic villus sampling

Chorionic villus sampling (CVS) should not be offered routinely to women with epilepsy but restricted to the same indications as in women without epilepsy, i.e. a family history of chromosomal disorders or previous birth of an infant with chromosomal disease.

Amniocentesis

The standard amniocentesis is carried out at week 15–16 of gestation. The puncture of the amniotic sac is performed transabdominally. Ultrasound needle guidance is used, with a guideline shown on the VDU screen visualizing the position of the needle. A volume of 15–20 ml of amniotic fluid is aspirated for cytogenetic and biochemical examination. Due to the culture period of the amniotic fluid cells the reporting time of the chromosomal analysis is two to three weeks. Standard amniocentesis has been found to give an increased risk of spontaneous abortion of 1% and an increased incidence of respiratory distress syndrome and pneumonia in newborns. A few per cent of women exposed to amniocentesis will experience a minor vaginal escape of amniotic fluid for one or two days after the procedure. This is seldom of significance (Tabor et al., 1986).

An increased concentration of alpha-fetoprotein in the amniotic fluid (and in maternal serum) is found in cases of neural tube defects such as anencephaly, spina bifida and meningomyelocele, especially if not skin-covered. Furthermore, the amnion alpha-fetoprotein concentration is elevated in cases of abdominal wall defects. This malformation is not especially connected with epilepsy or antiepileptic drugs.

In order to decrease the gestational age at which the cytogenetic result is available, studies of the safety and the diagnostic accuracy of early amniocentesis are currently undertaken. Early amniocentesis is defined as amniocentesis before week 14 and as early as week 11 (Sundberg *et al.*, 1995). As the amount of amniotic fluid in week 12 is limited to 30–50 ml special techniques for sampling of amniotic cells have been developed. Furthermore, early amniocentesis will have to be evaluated and compared with standard amniocentesis with respect to fetal loss, cytogenetic results, and amnion alpha-fetoprotein. A recent report estimates fetal loss to be increased by 1% after early amniocentesis, i.e. the same level as after standard amniocentesis. The preliminary results seem to indicate that significantly elevated amnion alpha-fetoprotein concentrations are demonstrated in cases of fetal neural tube and abdominal wall defects. In standard amniocentesis the sensitivity of amnion AFP is greater than 98% (Jørgensen *et al.*, 1995).

Ultrasound examination at week 18–20

Pregnant women with epilepsy should be offered ultrasound examination at the gestational ages of 18–20 weeks and 33–34 weeks. The first examination offers the opportunity to detect malformations in the fetus, the second to be aware of signs of intrauterine growth retardation.

Routinely the examination is carried out transabdominally but the development of transvaginal sonography may demonstrate ability to detect malformations at an earlier gestational age.

The early ultrasound examination is claimed to have a high sensitivity (avoiding false-negative cases) and high specificity (avoiding false-positive cases) with values in the range of 85–100%, depending on the organ system. Sensitivity in detecting malformations of the gastrointestinal tract and the urinary system is lower (20–50%) than in detecting central nervous system malformations. Cardiac defects may be detected by including a four-chamber view in the examination.

The central nervous system

The most common malformation of the central nervous system is failure of the cranial part of the neural tube to close. There are geographical variations of the frequency. It results in acrania without formation of the parietal, frontal and occipital bones. The developed, protruding nervous tissue (exencephaly) will become necrotic, resulting in anencephaly. A more caudal failure of closure of the neural tube may be presented as an occipital cephalocele with a defect of the calvarium and further caudal as a meningocele or a meningomyelocele. There are spinal defects of different types and spina bifida is the generally used term.

The ultrasonographic diagnosis is based upon the typical echogenicity of the bony tissue, the skull and vertebrae. As ossification is not completed until after week 12, the diagnosis can hardly be achieved earlier than in the late first trimester (van Zalen-Sprock *et al.*, 1994).

The cardiovascular system

The four-chamber view of the heart includes the two atria and the two ventricles, which in pairs are of approximately equal size. The heart occupies about one-third of the fetal thorax. Furthermore, the atrioventricular valves are observed. Reported figures of sensitivity vary from 36–77% depending on the prevalence of congenital heart disease and the gestational age at examination, which should not be less than 18 weeks. Where echocardiographic equipment and experts are available the sensitivity in recognizing cardiac malformations is 80% at a later gestational age (week 24) (Mandruzzato *et al.*, 1994).

At the early ultrasound examination it should be possible to reveal such anomalies as ventricular septal defects, the tetralogy of Fallot, single ventricle or hypoplastic ventricle.

The skeletal system and oral clefts

Normal growth of the fetal skeleton has been studied from week 12 onwards and it is possible at the early examinations to detect skeletal dysplasia. At this time the digits are delineated. Abnormalities such as polydactyly or club foot may be demonstrated.

Facial deformities, such as cleft lip and palate, should be able to be visualized from week 16. The recent introduction of three-dimensional ultrasonography may lead to an improvement in the diagnosis of facial defects. By this technique astonishingly detailed images of the fetal facial features are obtained as well as of hand and foot at week 20 (Jurkovic *et al.*, 1994).

The urinary tract

The fetal kidneys have reached their adult shape and position by week 10–12. Filling of the bladder may be observed from this time. Failure to demonstrate the bladder in the early second trimester may be a sign of a defective urinary tract. An enlarged fetal bladder appearing as a large cystic mass in the fetal abdomen indicates a bladder outlet obstruction. Failure of bladder filling is a finding combined with nonfunctional polycystic kidneys or aplasia of the kidneys. Especially in the latter half of pregnancy it will be accompanied by oligohydramnios. Hydronephrosis may be transient and disappear, but can persist and be detected as early as week 13–16.

The gastrointestinal tract

Abdominal wall defects cannot be diagnosed until after week 12 as a physiological umbilical herniation may still be seen in normal developing fetuses. An omphalocele is very often (75%) associated with other anomalies (van Zalen-Sprock *et al.*, 1994). Congenital diaphragmatic hernias may be visualized as a stomach bubble in the chest of the fetus. The condition may be complicated by pulmonary hypoplasia. Intestinal atresia may be demonstrated by recognizable dilatation of the intestinal tract oral to the obstruction, especially at a later stage of gestation.

INTRAUTERINE GROWTH RETARDATION

Intrauterine growth retardation (IUGR) is defined as an impairment of the fetal growth potential *in utero* and may be detected by serial ultrasound determinations at intervals of 12–14 days. The fetal weight gain will be less than expected compared with the reference values. It is a sign of fetal distress and malnutrition. However, an infant of a birthweight low for the gestational age (below the fifth or tenth percentile) is not necessarily growth-retarded. It may be of low birthweight for genetic, constitutional reasons (Carrera and Mallafré, 1994).

IUGR has been reported as a complication in pregnancies of women with epilepsy and is one of the three major problems in obstetrics today, the others being fetal malformations and preterm births. There is a wide range of maternal and fetal factors in the aetiology of IUGR. Chronic maternal disease involving vascular or renal impairment is well known. Fetal chromosome abnormalities, inherited syndromes, or fetal infections are other factors which may be recognized in some cases of IUGR. Mostly it must be concluded that the cause of growth retardation is not known or due to malfunction of the uteroplacental unit. The consequences of IUGR for the infant can be perinatal asphyxia and increased long-term morbidity with abnormal behaviour patterns and neurological deficits.

The growth of the fetus at the early stage of gestation is assessed by measuring the crown–rump length from week 6–14. The gestational age is in 95% of cases estimated with an error not greater than plus or minus five days.

The biparietal diameter is measured from the fourteenth week of gestation. It is a most reproducible parameter. The biparietal diameter increases linearly until week 30, with a weekly increment of 3 mm. From week 30 the rate of change gradually slows. The fetal abdominal diameter (or the abdominal circumference) is assessed at the same time and the fetal weight is read from a nomogram based on a line drawn between the values of the two diameters. Weeks 32–34 are considered to be the best time for differentiating fetuses with IUGR.

A prerequisite for the diagnosis of IUGR in the third trimester is early assessment (at week 16–18) of the biparietal diameter predicting the estimated date of delivery plus or minus seven days.

FUTURE ASPECTS

For obvious reasons efforts are being aimed at a diagnosis of congenital malformations at the earliest time of pregnancy. This goal will probably be achieved by early amniocentesis before week 14. The refinement of the techniques for transvaginal and three-dimensional ultrasonography shows promise in detecting serious disorders at an early stage. Chorionic villus sampling, combined with the development in DNA technology in mapping genes, could be of consequence in the context of epilepsy and pregnancy.

REFERENCES

Carrera, J.M. and Mallafré, J. (1994). Intrauterine growth retardation. In: Kurjak, A. and Chervenak, F.A. (Eds), *The Fetus as a Patient*. Parthenon Publishing, London, pp. 251–287.

Delgado-Escueta, A.V. and Janz, D. (1992). Consensus guidelines: preconception counseling, management, and care of the pregnant woman with epilepsy. *Neurology* **42** (suppl 5), 149–160.

Jørgensen, F.S. (1995). Declining an alpha-fetoprotein test in pregnancy, why and who? *Acta Obstet Gynecol Scand* **74**, 3–11.

Jørgensen, F.S., Sundberg, K., Loft, A.G.R., Arends, J. and Nørgaard-Pedersen, B. (1995). Alpha-fetoprotein and acetylcholinesterase activity in first- and early second-trimester amniotic fluid. *Prenat Diagn* **15**, 621–625.

Jurkovic, D., Jauniaux, E. and Campbell, S. (1994). Three-dimensional ultrasound in obstetrics and gynecology. In: Kurjak, A. and Chervenak, F.A. (Eds), *The Fetus as a Patient*. Parthenon Publishing, London, pp. 135–140.

Källén, B. (1986). A register study of maternal epilepsy and delivery outcome with special reference to drug use. *Acta Neurol Scand* **73**, 253–259.

Kaneko, S., Otani, K., Fukushima, Y. *et al.* (1988). Teratogenicity of antiepileptic drugs: analysis of possible risk factors. *Epilepsia* **29**, 459–467.

Kjessler, B. and Johansson, S.G.D. (1977). Monitoring of the development of early pregnancy by determination of alpha-fetoprotein in maternal serum and amniotic fluid samples. *Acta Obstet Gynecol Scand* **56** (suppl 69), 5–14.

Lindhout, D. and Schmidt, D. (1986). *In utero* exposure to valproate and neural-tube defects. *Lancet* **ii**, 1932.

Lindhout, D., Hoppener, R.J.E.A. and Meinardi, H. (1984). Teratogenicity of antiepileptic drug combinations with special emphasis on epoxidation of carbamazepine. *Epilepsia* **25**, 77–83.

Mandruzzato, G.P., D'Ottavio, G. and Rustico, M.A. (1994). Screening with ultrasound in obstetrics. In: Kurjak, A. and Chervenak, F.A. (Eds), *The Fetus as a Patient*. Parthenon Publishing, London, pp. 57–69.

Nørgaard-Pedersen, B., Bagger, P., Bang, J. *et al.* (1985). Maternal-serum-alphafeto-protein screening for fetal malformations in 28 062 pregnancies. *Acta Obstet Gynecol Scand* **64**, 511–514.

Report of the RCOG Working Party on Biochemical Markers and the Detection of Down's Syndrome (1993). The Royal College of Obstetricians and Gynaecologists, London.

Sundberg, K.L., Jørgensen, F.S., Tabor, A. and Bang, J. (1995). Experience with early amniocentesis. *J Perinat Med* **23**, 149–158.

Tabor, A., Philip, J., Madsen, M., Bang, J., Obel, E.B. and Nørgaard-Pedersen, B. (1986). Randomised controlled trial of genetic amniocentesis in 4606 low-risk women. *Lancet* **i**, 1287.

van Zalen-Sprock, M.M., van Vugt, J.M.G. and van Geiju, H.P. (1994). Early detection of congenital anomalies using ultrasonography. In: Kurjak, A. and Chervenak, F.A. (Eds), *The Fetus as a Patient*. Parthenon Publishing, London, pp. 127–134.

Vestermark, V. (1993). Teratogenicity of carbamazepine: a review of the literature. *Dev Brain Dysfunct* **6**, 266–278.

Epilepsy and Pregnancy
Edited by T. Tomson, L. Gram, M. Sillanpää and S.I. Johannessen
© 1997 Wrightson Biomedical Publishing Ltd

15

Genetic Aspects of Malformations

MOGENS LAUE FRIIS

Department of Neurology, Odense University Hospital, Odense, Denmark

INTRODUCTION

Few drugs have been scrutinized for possible teratogenic effects as thoroughly as antiepileptic drugs (AEDs). Much uncertainty remains concerning the risks of fetotoxicity linked to individual AEDs and which drugs are strong and which are weak teratogens. These questions are extremely relevant to both the physician and the patient. The problem is increasing as most major epidemiological investigations (case–control or cohort studies) on AED teratology have been carried out on the older AEDs such as phenobarbital (PB), phenytoin (PHT) and primidone (PRM) (Kelly, 1984; Friis, 1989). Some good studies on carbamazepine (CBZ) and valproic acid (VPA) have been published, whereas our knowledge of the use of 'newer' AEDs such as oxcarbazepine (OXC), lamotrigine (LTG), gabapentine (GPT), topiramate (TPM), felbamate (FBM) and experimental drugs is limited or nonexistent. In this context a relevant problem is that the use of new and experimental AEDs in pregnancy and in women of childbearing age wanting to have children is restricted. Therefore our knowledge on the possible teratogenicity of the new AEDs will be based on accidental pregnancies voluntarily reported to either central regulatory agencies or to pharmaceutical companies, with the risk of severe selection and ascertainment bias in the databases. One in every 250–300 newborns has been exposed to one or more AEDs during the first trimester of pregnancy. From the literature, the risk of a major malformation in these AED-exposed children is about 7–10% (Friis, 1989; Lindhout and Omtzigt, 1992). In Denmark, with approximately 5.2 million inhabitants and approximately 50 000 newborns per year, this means that, in a conservative estimate, 200 newborns are exposed to AEDs prenatally and that 14–20 children each year are born with a major malformation such as cleft lip with or without cleft palate (CL(P)), cleft palate (CP), congenital heart defect (CHD), neural tube defect (NTD), or skeletal or urogenital malformations attributable to AEDs.

HISTORICAL BACKGROUND

AEDs were focused on as teratogens when Müller-Küppers (1963) reported on an AED-exposed malformed child with a cleft palate and other defects. One year later Janz and Fuchs (1964) studied 358 children of mothers with epilepsy; 225 of these were born to AED-treated mothers with epilepsy. They found that only five children had malformations and concluded that AEDs were not a serious risk factor regarding congenital malformations. A detailed analysis of the individual malformations reported, however, suggests that the risk of CL(P)/CP is increased approximately five- to sixfold compared with background population values.

Meadow (1968) found that surprisingly many children born with facial clefts had mothers with epilepsy. Several studies (Dronamraju, 1970; Pashayan et al., 1971; Erickson and Oakley, 1974) subsequently all found a higher frequency of maternal epilepsy among children born with facial clefts.

In the early studies of malformation, epilepsy and anticonvulsant drugs, teratogenicity was emphasized. Later a possible genetic association between epilepsy and the malformations in question was explored (Kelly, 1984; Friis, 1989).

FACIAL CLEFTS

CL(P)/CP are among the most frequent congenital malformations with an incidence of one to two cases per 1000 newborns. Several studies have suggested that maternal epilepsy is a risk factor for the development of CL(P)/CP in children. However, it is evident that there is a strong genetic component in the aetiology of these major malformations (Fogh-Andersen, 1942). Annegers et al. (1974) and Shapiro et al. (1976) found indications that paternal epilepsy also could increase the risk of congenital malformations in the offspring, whereas no specific evidence was found of an increased CL(P)/CP risk. Friis et al. (1979) reported on maternal and paternal epilepsy and AED exposure among 391 live-born children with CL(P) or CP. Eighteen persons with epilepsy (7 fathers and 11 mothers) were identified. The point prevalence of epilepsy among parents of CL(P)/CP patients is thus 2.3% or around three times the expected value, with no statistical difference between the number of fathers and mothers with epilepsy. The pattern of AED treatment was no different from expectation and thus the result suggested that epilepsy *per se* could play a role in the genesis of CL(P)/CP in the offspring of patients with epilepsy. We and others investigated this issue in further detail. Kelly et al. (1984) found 13 parents, 11 mothers and 2 fathers, with epilepsy of 175 probands with isolated CL(P) and no instances of parental epilepsy among 140 probands with other cleft-ing than CL(P), including isolated CP. In a case–control study of drug exposure conducted by Greenberg *et al.* (1977) an increased exposure to phenobarbital was found among 412 malformed infants with CL(P)/CP. However, the statistical significance of the phenobarbital correlation was lost when mothers with a close family history of birth defects were excluded. Friis *et al.* (1981) identified 11 patients with facial clefts among 3 203 epilep-tics, whereas only five were expected using Danish incidence figures, supporting an association between facial clefts and epilepsy *per se*. These results indicate that, when a child with CL(P)/CP is born following first trimester exposure to one or more AEDs, a thorough family history on CL(P)/CP should be taken (Friis *et al.*, 1986). It is important not to rule out the possibility of using an otherwise relevant and effective AED. Furthermore, the genetics of facial clefts needs further investigation, and genetic methods will possibly elucidate this issue in the future.

CONGENITAL HEART DEFECTS

Anderson (1976) was one of the first to report on an increased incidence of CHD in the offspring of AED-treated mothers with epilepsy. He found 18 cases of maternal epilepsy amongst approximately 3 000 new paediatric patients with CHD seen at the University of Minnesota Hospital from 1961 to 1975. He reported on an increased rate of CHD in children prenatally exposed to AEDs; however, if those children exposed to known, severe teratogens such as trimethadione and paramethadione, and those patients giving rise to the study are excluded (a total of four and three patients, respectively, or, combined, six patients), the CHD incidence is approximately 12 : 2 400 or 1 : 200 which is lower or closer to expectation in most countries with efficient malformation registries. Anderson (1976) found that these 18 children of mothers with epilepsy had a wide range of different CHDs. However, he noted that an apparent skewing of the distribution towards ventricular septal defects and pulmonary stenosis in combination with other congenital malformations could suggest a malformation specificity involving these two CHDs. No study with more patients with CHD has been published since. Friis and Hauge (1985) found no increase of CHDs in children of either mothers or fathers with epilepsy. However, the genetics of CHDs (e.g. Steno-Fallot's tetralogy) is even more complicated than that of CL(P)/CP; here also future genetic studies may help to elucidate some of these issues. Epidemiological studies have reached a magnitude where international co-operation is certainly needed if future problems on epilepsy, AEDs and malformations, including CHD, are to be solved using ordinary epidemio-logical methods.

NEURAL TUBE DEFECTS

NTDs are also influenced by both environmental and genetic factors. Robert and Guibaud (1982), in their first publication on valproate teratogenicity, noted that three of nine NTD infants had a relative with spina bifida. Later, Lindhout et al. (1992a) and Rosa (1991) also presented evidence that carbamazepine was associated with NTD, although not as strongly as valproate. Lindhout et al. (1992b) analysed the spectrum of NTDs in 34 infants prenatally exposed to AEDs (preferably valproate and carbamazepine). They found an anencephaly to lumbosacral spina bifida aperta ratio of 1 : 33, suggesting a specific association with caudal CNS defects. Other midline defects were also associated with valproate (hypospadias (two), hypertelorism (two), partial agenesis of the corpus callosum, agenesis of septum pellucidum with lissencephaly of the mesial sides of the occipital lobes, Dandy–Walker anomaly and CHD). However, no specific association with either maternal family history of NTDs or epilepsy was found. Klepel and Freitag (1992) examined 182 children and adolescents with epilepsy aged 3–18 years for the presence of closed spina bifida. They found, in contrast to the background population, that sacral localization was predominant among epilepsy patients and that patients with idiopathic epilepsy had the highest frequency of spina bifida, suggesting an association between closed sacral spina bifida and idiopathic epilepsy. However, no statistically significant differences were found in this particular study, probably due to the small sample size.

CONCLUSION

In the counselling of patients with epilepsy needing AEDs it is important to know whether there is a genetic relationship between epilepsy and birth defects. Previously published epidemiological studies have neither proven nor excluded an association between any disease or syndrome with epilepsy and an individual congenital malformation. However, molecular genetics in the future will be able to localize both the genes for selected congenital defects such as CL(P) and the major epilepsy syndromes such as juvenile myoclonic epilepsy, thus elucidating some of the issues reviewed here. Likewise, the rapid development in pharmacogenetics may give some clues. An example of how geneticists in collaboration with clinicians have elucidated the influence of genetic background on the fetal hydantoin syndrome is given by Phelan et al. (1982). They reported on an Afro-American woman giving birth to heteropaternal dizygotic twins, showing marked differences with regard to the different components of the fetal hydantoin syndrome. Twin A had poor growth and a broad, depressed nasal bridge, whereas twin

B, in addition, had mild mental retardation, brachycephaly, characteristic facial appearance with hypertelorism and wide mouth with prominent lips, and also small nails and rib abnormality. Although dizygotic twins are normally assumed to be as similar genetically as ordinary siblings, the members of this set of twins had only one parent in common, and are thus related as half-siblings. The discordant expression of the fetal hydantoin syndrome in this pair of heteropaternal twins exposed to the same concentrations of phenytoin for approximately the same time period provides evidence that the genetic sensitivity of the fetus is a relevant factor in the embryopathic effect of AEDs.

Finally it is emphasized that in any case of congenital minor anomaly or major malformation, or of mental retardation following maternal AED treatment, it should be mandatory to perform thorough paediatric, teratologic and genetic analysis of the affected child and its family. Causes other than prenatal exposure to AEDs must be ruled out in order to determine the recurrence risk and to institute therapy where termination of later pregnancies is the extreme option.

REFERENCES

Anderson, R.C. (1976). Cardiac defects in children of mothers receiving anticonvulsant therapy during pregnancy. *J Pediatr* **89**, 318–319.

Annegers, J.F., Elveback, L.R., Hauser, W.A. and Kurland, L.T. (1974). Do anticonvulsants have a teratogenic effect? *Arch Neurol* **31**, 364–373.

Dronamraju, K.R. (1970). Epilepsy and cleft lip and palate. *Lancet* **ii**, 876–877.

Erickson, J.D. and Oakley, G.P. (1974). Seizure disorder in mothers of children with orofacial clefts: a case–control study. *J Pediatr* **84**, 244–246.

Fogh-Andersen, P. (1942). Inheritance of harelip and cleft palate (Thesis). Nyt Nordisk Forlag, Arnold Busck, Copenhagen.

Friis, M.L. (1979). Epilepsy among parents of children with facial clefts. *Epilepsia* **20**, 69–76.

Friis, M.L. (1989). Facial clefts and congenital heart defects in children of parents with epilepsy: genetic and environmental etiologic factors. *Acta Neurol Scand* **79**, 433–459.

Friis, M.L. and Hauge, M. (1985). Congenital heart defects in live-born children of epileptic parents. *Arch Neurol* **42**, 374–376.

Friis, M.L., Broeng-Nielsen, B., Sindrup, E.H., Lund, M., Fogh-Andersen, P. and Hauge, M. (1981). Facial clefts among epileptic patients. *Arch Neurol* **38**, 227–229.

Friis, M.L., Holm, N.V., Sindrup, E.H., Fogh-Andersen, P. and Hauge, M. (1986). Facial clefts in sibs and children of epileptic patients. *Neurology* **36**, 346–350.

Greenberg, G., Inman, W.H.W., Weatherall, J.A.C., Adelstein, A.M. and Haskey, J.C. (1977). Maternal drug histories and congenital abnormalities. *BMJ* **2**, 853–856.

Janz, D. and Fuchs, U. (1964). Sind antiepileptische Medikamente während der Schwangerschaft schädlich? *Dtsch Med Wochenschr* **89**, 241–243.

Kelly, T.E. (1984). Teratogenicity of anticonvulsant drugs I: review of the literature. *Am J Med Genet* **19**, 413–434.

Kelly, T.E., Rein, M. and Edwards, P. (1984). Teratogenicity of anticonvulsant drugs IV. The association of clefting and epilepsy. *Am J Med Genet* **19**, 451–458.

Klepel, H. and Freitag, G. (1992). Spina bifida occulta in epilepsy syndromes. *Neurology* **42** (suppl 5), 126–127.

Lindhout, D. and Omtzigt, J.G.C. (1992). Pregnancy and the risk of teratogenicity. *Epilepsia* **33** (suppl 4), 41–48.

Lindhout, D., Meinardi, H., Meijer, J.W.A. and Nau, H. (1992a). Antiepileptic drugs and teratogenesis in two consecutive cohorts: changes in prescription policy paralleled by change in pattern of malformations. *Neurology* **42** (suppl 5), 94–110.

Lindhout, D., Omtzigt, J.G.C. and Cornel, M.C. (1992b). Spectrum of neural tube defects in 34 infants prenatally exposed to antiepileptic drugs. *Neurology* **42** (suppl 5), 111–118.

Meadow, S.R. (1968). Anticonvulsant drugs and congenital abnormalities. *Lancet* **ii**, 1296.

Müller-Küppers, M. (1963). Zur Frage der Fruchtschädigung in der Schwangerschaft durch Einnahme von Antieptileptika. *Acta Paedopsychiatr* **30**, 401–405.

Pashayan, H., Pruzansky, D. and Pruzansky, S. (1971). Are anticonvulsants teratogenic? *Lancet* **ii**, 702–703.

Phelan, M.C., Pellock, J.M. and Nance, W.E. (1982). Discordant expression of fetal hydantoin syndrome in heteropaternal dizygotic twins. *N Engl J Med* **307**, 99–101.

Robert, E. and Guibaud, P. (1982). Maternal valproic acid and congenital neural tube defects. *Lancet* **ii**, 937.

Rosa, F.W. (1991). Spina bifida in infants of women treated with carbamazepine during pregnancy. *N Engl J Med* **324**, 674–677.

Shapiro, S., Slone, D., Hartz, S.C. *et al.* (1976). Anticonvulsants and parental epilepsy in the development of birth defects. *Lancet* **i**, 272–275.

Epilepsy and Pregnancy
Edited by T. Tomson, L. Gram, M. Sillanpää and S.I. Johannessen
© 1997 Wrightson Biomedical Publishing Ltd

16

The Molecular Background of Human Disease

LEENA PELTONEN

*National Public Health Institute and Institute of Biomedicine,
University of Helsinki, Helsinki, Finland*

THE CURRENT STATUS OF THE GENOME PROGRAMME

The mapping and characterization of the human genome have progressed with increasing speed over the past two decades. The current version of the map contains over 5000 highly polymorphic markers which can efficiently and with high certainty be identified from individuals' DNA samples and utilized as tools to assign disease genes to specific locations (defined chromosomal regions) of the genome. The sets of ordered markers on individual chromosomes form the *genetic* map of the human genome (Dib *et al.*, 1996).

As the next step of the genome-mapping effort, wide chromosomal DNA regions are already being cloned in vectors which can accommodate large-size inserts, facilitating identification, ordering and orientation of individual genes. These clones represent the *physical* map of the human genome and, although not hole-proof at this point, they already cover a distinct majority of DNA of all chromosomes (Chumakov *et al.*, 1995; Hudson *et al.*, 1995). The large clones of the physical map serve as targets for large-scale sequencing efforts and also for efforts to create transcript maps. Several groups have contributed to the production of tissue-specific 'expressed sequence tags' (ESTs) by producing short sequences from random cDNAs reverse-transcribed from RNA extracted from a given tissue (Adams *et al.*, 1991). When these ESTs are positioned on long-range physical clones they form a *transcript map* of the human genome. Hundreds of thousands of ESTs already exist in databases, so some information actually exists on some 70 000 human genes – just like letters from complex gene-words (Fields *et al.*, 1994). However, only a fraction of ESTs are so far well positioned either in genetic

Human Genome Project:
(stage completed)

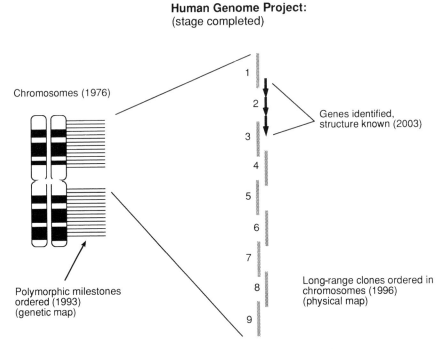

Figure 1. Schematic presentation of the maturation stages of human genome maps. From long band-stained chromosomes in the 1970s the precision of the genome map has progressed to well ordered physical clones for most chromosomes in 1996 and aims at identification of all of about 70 000 genes by 2003.

or in physical maps of individual chromosomes (Boguski and Schuler, 1995; IMAGE database, 1996).

This set of tools, comprising genetic maps constructed from polymorphic milestones separated by less than one million basepairs on average, physical maps consisting of individual clones up to 500 000 bp in size, and transcript maps, are all planned and manufactured thanks to the Human Genome Project (schematically presented in Figure 1). The efficient utilization of these tools will eventually lead to isolation and detailed characterization of all human disease genes. Once the genes behind diseases have been identified, they will serve as tools for dissection of the molecular pathogenesis of individual diseases. In this short review, the steps involved in the process are described, from identification of the disease locus to an understanding of the molecular details of the cellular and tissue events disturbed by the disease mutation. Examples of different steps are taken from our own research.

ASSIGNMENT OF DISEASE LOCI

Over 200 inherited disease loci have been positioned on well defined chromosomal regions without any previous knowledge of their structure or function (Genome database, 1996). The positioning is based on the analysis of polymorphic markers of the genetic map in family or sibpair, or population materials containing a high number of affected individuals. Whenever the affected individuals have inherited the same marker alleles more often than expected by chance, this suggests that the disease locus is close to this particular marker. The sharing of the same marker alleles is statistically evaluated using linkage-based analysis (in families) or non-linkage-based analysis in sibpairs or association materials. The assignment of a disease locus is especially feasible in isolated populations with one or only a few founder mutations. If the majority of affected individuals are descendants of the same founder individual, first affected by the mutation, they will still share a relatively wide DNA region flanking the mutation and reflecting the outlook of the ancient chromosome, the target of the ancestor mutation. Such a region is easy to identify, even with a relatively sparse set of polymorphic markers, whereas much more numerous markers must be tested in more mixed populations (Peltonen et al., 1995).

This is well exemplified by our mapping of the infantile-onset spinocerebellar ataxia (IOSCA) locus by primary screening of the genome using samples from just four affected individuals in two consanguineous families. The primary random screen of the genome was made by genotyping the four affected individuals followed by simple eyeballing for shared marker genotypes. Only these chromosomal regions were examined further, first by genotyping the complete family set by using the markers in question, and then by carrying out conventional linkage analysis. We initially scanned 213 polymorphic DNA markers scattered at ~20 cM distances throughout the genome using the samples of these four patients. Of these markers, only two showed similar genotypes in these related individuals. Linkage analysis of the complete family material excluded one of the loci as the chromosomal region for IOSCA, whereas the other revealed evidence for linkage (Nikali et al., 1995).

FROM ASSIGNMENT OF DISEASE LOCUS TO IDENTIFICATION OF MUTATION

Although hundreds of disease loci have been mapped onto individual chromosomes, the process resulting in the final identification of the disease gene is still relatively slow. This is reflected by the fact that only some 40 genes have been conclusively isolated based on this strategy, known as positional cloning (Collins, 1995). In practice, scientists still have to analyse in detail large DNA clones in the chromosomal region where markers indicate the position of the disease locus. If they are lucky, some well characterized genes will already exist in the region and can be immediately tested as potential disease genes (sequenced through in patients). More often, scientists still have to look for novel coding regions by adopting multiple strategies in order to find all genes in the critical DNA region. When testing whether known genes fall in this DNA region, or when ordering and positioning novel DNA regions, we have been greatly helped by the recently developed spectrum of different visual mapping strategies. These methods facilitate visual ordering of individual clones via a relatively rapid and simple process (Heiskanen *et al.*, 1996) (Figure 2). This is well exemplified by our recent identification of the defective gene in the severe brain disorder of children, infantile neuronal ceroid lipofuscinosis (INCL). Visual inspection of fluorescent signals of clones known to flank the critical DNA region and of a novel, recently identified gene indicated that this gene was situated in the middle of our critical DNA region. Sequence analysis then identified

Visual mapping of genes by FISH (Fluorescent *in situ* hybridization)

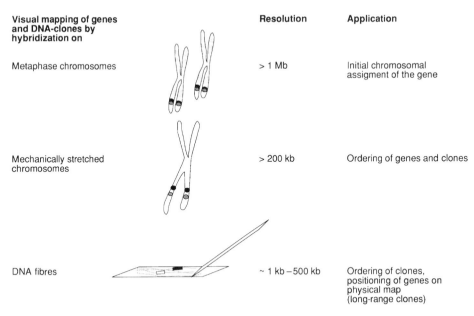

Visual mapping of genes and DNA-clones by hybridization on	Resolution	Application
Metaphase chromosomes	> 1 Mb	Initial chromosomal assigment of the gene
Mechanically stretched chromosomes	> 200 kb	Ordering of genes and clones
DNA fibres	~ 1 kb – 500 kb	Ordering of clones, positioning of genes on physical map (long-range clones)

Figure 2. Visual mapping and ordering of clones and genes has greatly facilitated the construction of high-density maps on individual chromosomes. In this method different resolution levels can be obtained by the use of hybridization targets representing different condensation levels of chromosomal DNA.

mutations in INCL patients in this gene encoding palmitoyl protein thioesterase, a new lysosomal enzyme (Vesa *et al.*, 1995).

FROM MUTATION TO MOLECULAR PATHOGENESIS

Once the disease gene has been identified, the cloned gene facilitates detailed functional analysis of the normal and mutated gene product. The wild type cDNA and *in vitro* mutagenized cDNA mimicking the human disease mutation can be transfected into cultured cells and expressed there *in vitro*. The fate of normal and diseased protein inside the cell can then be followed by pulse chase experiments and immunological analysis (Figure 3).

In our *in vitro* experiments dissecting the cellular consequences of the INCL mutation, the wild type protein is transported to lysosomes and serves its function: removal of palmitoyl residues from palmitoylated proteins in this cellular destination. The mutated protein, changed by one amino acid only, is retained in the endoplasmic reticulum and degraded there (Figure 4)

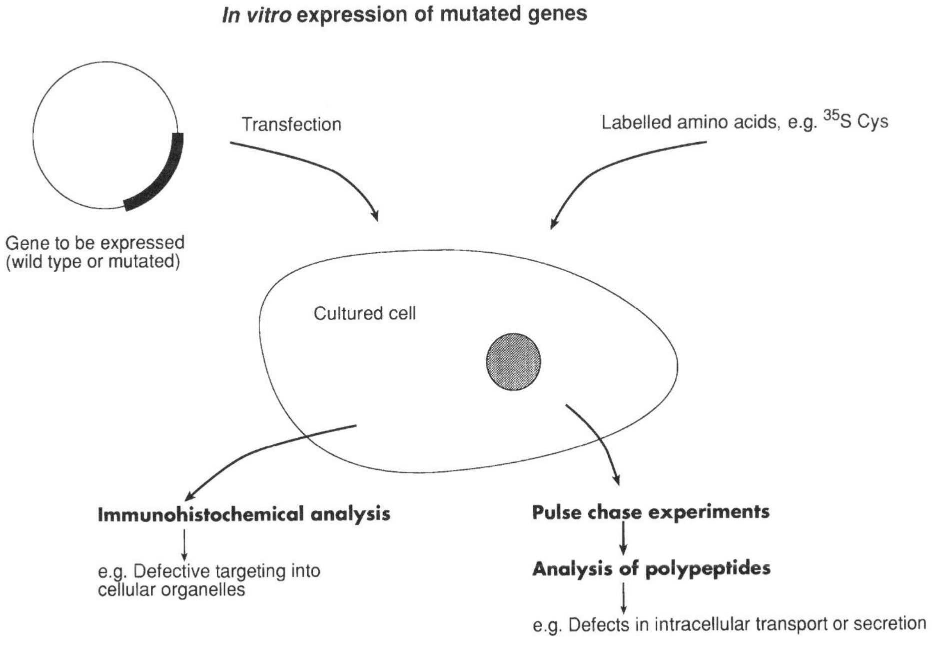

Figure 3. The cellular consequences of identified disease mutations can be monitored by expressing the genes of interest in cultured cells. The fate of normal (wild-type) and mutated gene product can be followed by biochemical and immunological analysis.

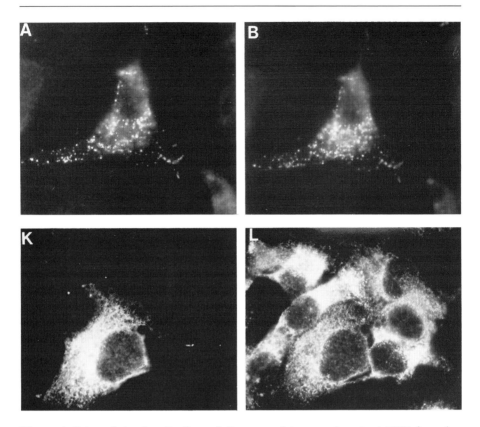

Figure 4. Intracellular localization of the normal type and mutant PPT (carrying INCL-Fin mutation) in transiently transfected COS-1 cells after blocking the continuous protein synthesis by cycloheximide. The staining pattern of the wild-type PPT (A) is characteristic for lysosomal staining (B) visualized with antibody against B-hexosaminidase whereas the mutated PPT is retained in the endoplasmic reticulum (K) visualized with antibody against KDEL (Lys-Asp-Glu-Leu)-motif, characteristic for ER proteins. (Adapted from Hellsten *et al.*, 1996).

(Hellsten *et al.*, 1996). Consequently, the enzyme cannot reach its functional location and the cells accumulate non-cleaved palmitoylated peptides which disturb their life (being especially fatal for cortical neurons).

The identification of defects in intracellular transport or handling of the mutated protein does not necessarily provide the final explanation for molecular pathogenesis. Information is also needed on the precise structure of the protein, defective in disease. The major drug companies invest large amounts in this area since it provides the basis for targeted, tailor-made therapies utilizing correctly modelled molecules. We have been analysing the molecular defect in aspartylglucosaminuria (AGU) which results in severe mental retardation and is caused by mutations in the gene encoding aspartylglucosaminidase, also a lysosomal enzyme. We have crystallized the enzyme molecule and, by X-ray diffraction analysis, determined the three-dimensional structure of this catalytically active protein. All amino acids necessary for active site formation and enzyme catalysis were identified and the defect caused by the major AGU mutation into this structure was characterized (Ikonen *et al.*, 1991; Oinonen *et al.*, 1995). This information provided new knowledge for future developments of substitution therapy in this severe disease.

Conclusive information on tissue consequences of disease mutations can be obtained only via genetically modified animals carrying disease mutations in their genome. For research purposes the genetically engineered animals are produced by two strategies: either by bringing the disease gene into intact mouse genome (transgenic animals) or by replacing the corresponding mouse gene with defective human gene (knock-out animals). The transgenic mice characteristically serve as models for dominantly inherited diseases and the knock-out mice for recessive diseases. These animals facilitate monitoring of the tissue-specific symptoms of disease during development and ageing and also provide essential targets for various therapeutic trials. We have produced an AGU mouse which carries the AGU mutation (detection of one exon) in both maternal and paternal alleles. The consequences of disease mutation can now be carefully monitored in the brain cells of this mouse, an experiment which is impossible to perform in humans. This genetically engineered mouse is also an ideal target for both traditional substitution therapy with the enzyme protein as well as for gene therapy trials in future.

Only after careful analysis of all these experimental models can scientists claim to have dissected the details of molecular pathogenesis of a human disease caused by a mutation identified in affected individuals, and only then is a solid basis built for rational developmental work towards focused therapy. Considering the cost, the professional skills and the multiple technologies required in this process, it is not an overstatement to claim that fruits of the Genome Project (cloned genes and identified disease mutations) will provide fuel for biomedical research for the next hundred years. Theoretically, by the year 2003, when all human genes should have been cloned, will we, for the first time in human history, have the precise tools with which to initiate our effort to characterize and understand the molecular basis of human diseases.

REFERENCES

Adams, M.D., Kelley, J.M., Gocayne, J.D. *et al.* (1991). Complementary DNA sequencing: expressed sequence tags and human Genome Project. *Science* **252**, 1651–1656.

Boguski, M.S. and Schuler, G.D. (1995). Establishing a human transcript map. *Nat Genet* **10**, 369–371.

Chumakov, I.M., Rigault, P. and Le Call, I. (1995). A YAC contig map of the human genome. *Nature* **28**, 175–183.

Collins, F.S. (1995). Positional cloning moves from perditional to traditional. *Nat Genet* **9**, 347–350.

Dib, C., Fauré, S., Fizames, C. *et al.* (1996). A comprehensive genetic map of the human genome based on 5264 microsatellites. *Nature* **380**, 152–154.

Fields, C., Adams, M.D., White, O. *et al.* (1994). How many genes in the human genome? *Nat Genet* **7**, 345–346.

Genome database (1996). http://gdbwww.gdb.org. and http://gdbwww.db.org/genomic_links.html.

Heiskanen, M., Peltonen, L. and Palotie, A. Visual mapping by high resolution FISH. *Trends Genet* 1997 (in press).

Hellsten, E., Vesa, J., Olkkonen, V.M. *et al.* (1996). Palmitoyl protein thioesterase: evidence for lysosomal targeting of the enzyme and disturbed processing in infantile neuronal ceroid lipofuscinosis. *EMBO* **15:18**, 5240–5245.

Hudson, T.J., Stein, L.D. *et al* (1995). An STS-based map of the human genome. *Science* **270**, 1945–1954.

Ikonen, E., Baumann, M., Grön, K. *et al.* (1991). Aspartylglucosaminuria: cDNA encoding human aspartylglucosaminidase and the missense mutation causing the disease. *EMBO* **10**, 51–58.

IMAGE (Integrated Molecular Analysis of Gene Expression) (1996). http://www-bio.llnl.gov/bbrp/genome/genome.html.

Nikali, K., Suomalainen, A., Terwilliger, J. *et al.* (1995). Random search for shared chromosomal regions in four affected individuals: the assignment of a new hereditary ataxia locus. *Am J Hum Genet* **56**, 1088–1095.

Oinonen, C., Tikkanen, R. and Rouvinen, J. (1995). Three-dimensional structure of human lysosomal aspartylglucosaminidase. *Nat Struct Biol* **2**, 1102–1107.

Peltonen, L., Pekkarinen, P. and Aaltonen, J. (1995). Messages from an isolate: lessons from the Finnish gene pool. *Biol Chem Hoppe-Seyler* **376**, 697–704.

Vesa, J., Hellsten, E., Verkruyse, L.-A. *et al.* (1995). Mutations in the palmitoyl protein thioesterase gene causing infantile neuronal ceroid lipofuscinosis. *Nature* **376**, 584–587.

Epilepsy and Pregnancy
Edited by T. Tomson, L. Gram, M. Sillanpää and S.I. Johannessen
© 1997 Wrightson Biomedical Publishing Ltd

17

Current Methods in Genetic Studies of Epilepsy

R. MARK GARDINER
Department of Paediatrics, University College London Medical School, London, UK

INTRODUCTION

Classical genetic studies over many years have clearly established a genetic aetiology of a number of human epilepsies and epilepsy syndromes and it has been estimated that in about one in five patients with epilepsy it has a genetic cause. Present research is directed towards an understanding of the genetic basis of human epilepsies at a molecular level. The aim is to identify the genes responsible, the proteins which they encode, and therefore to understand the mechanisms by which neuronal excitability is disturbed at a molecular level. A number of recent reviews of this field have been published (Bird, 1992; Dichter and Buchhalter, 1993; Leppert *et al.*, 1993; Rees and Gardiner, 1994).

The genetic epilepsies can be classified in a number of ways. Two important distinctions are the mode of inheritance – Mendelian or 'complex', non-Mendelian, and the distinction between 'pure' or 'idiopathic' epilepsies in which recurrent seizures occur in isolation, and those in which epilepsy occurs as one component of a more complex neurological or metabolic phenotype. In each case the two categories overlap.

There are over one hundred Mendelian conditions in which epilepsy occurs as part of a more complex phenotype. These include inborn errors of metabolism, neurodegenerative diseases, and neurocutaneous syndromes, for example, and the genes involved do not necessarily encode neuronal proteins. In addition, there are a few Mendelian 'pure' epilepsies, such as benign familial neonatal convulsions and autosomal dominant nocturnal frontal lobe epilepsy. In contrast, most 'idiopathic' epilepsies display a complex, non-Mendelian pattern of inheritance. These include conditions such as juvenile myoclonic epilepsy, idiopathic generalized epilepsy and the absence epilepsies. The latter account for a much larger number of patients than the Mendelian syndromes.

Three main strategies exist for the molecular genetic investigation of the inherited epilepsies. These strategies overlap to a very considerable extent and rely on the same molecular biological methodologies. They include gene mapping and 'positional cloning', candidate gene analysis and the investigation of animal models, especially in mice and rats.

In 'positional' cloning, co-segregation of the disease trait with any of a set of polymorphic DNA marker loci is sought in order to identify the map position of the disease gene. The location is subsequently refined in order to identify a chromosomal region small enough to allow the gene itself to be isolated. This approach is most easily applied to Mendelian disorders. In the second approach, cloned 'candidate' genes, in which a mutation might lead to the observed phenotype, are investigated by linkage analysis, population association studies, or direct sequence analysis. The last strategy involves the isolation of rodent epilepsy genes which may be homologous to similar disorders in man. These three strategies are considered in turn.

GENE MAPPING – POSITIONAL CLONING

The power of linkage analysis in investigation of human inherited diseases has been enormously enhanced by the construction of a high-resolution genetic map of the human genome. There are now several thousand 'microsatellite' marker loci on the human genetic map. The latest GENETHON human linkage map consists of 5264 short tandem (AC/TG) repeat polymorphisms with a mean heterozygosity of 70%. The average interval size is 1.6 cM, and only 1% remains in intervals above 10 cM.

Given an adequate family resource any genetically homogeneous Mendelian disorder can now be mapped. Individuals from families segregating the disease trait are typed using a set of DNA marker loci with the intention of finding 'linkage' – a marker locus which is inherited with the disease trait on account of its close proximity to the disease locus. The genome may be searched in a systematic way or priority may be given to genomic regions in which the likelihood of finding epilepsy genes is considered to be increased. Such regions may be identified because they harbour 'candidate' genes, they encompass cytogenetic aberrations associated with epilepsy, or because they correspond to genomic regions in the mouse to which murine epilepsy genes map.

This approach is most easily applied to autosomal dominant Mendelian disorders in which large multigenerational pedigrees are available. It can then be assumed that there is locus homogeneity. In autosomal recessive conditions data from numerous small nuclear pedigrees must be pooled and the existence of more than one locus causing the phenotype may render linkage difficult to establish.

Following the initial localization, additional families must be typed with a high-resolution map of marker loci in order to refine the localization to at least 1 cM. This corresponds to about 1 Mb of DNA which allows the implementation of 'end-stage' cloning procedures – construction of a physical map of the region, identification of transcripts (genes) and screening for mutations. The infrastructural information provided by the Human Genome Project has rendered this phase of the procedure much more tractable. It took 10 years from the initial localization to the isolation of the Huntington's disease gene. The existence of high-resolution genetic and physical maps for most of the genome is an enormous advantage, and when a complete gene map is available it will be possible to consult a computer database to identify candidate genes in a particular region.

Several Mendelian epilepsies have been mapped by linkage analysis. These include benign familial neonatal convulsions EBN1, EBN2 (Leppert *et al.*, 1989; Lewis *et al.*, 1993); Unverricht–Lundborg progressive myoclonic epilepsy EPM1 (Lehesjoki *et al.*, 1991); the neuronal ceroid lipofuscinoses CLN1, CLN3, CLN5; autosomal dominant frontal lobe epilepsy ADNFLE (Phillips *et al.*, 1995); partial epilepsy PE (Ottman *et al.*, 1995); and Lafora body disease LD (Serratosa *et al.*, 1995). Four of these are autosomal-dominant disease, and five are autosomal-recessive. Locus heterogeneity was found for benign familial neonatal convulsions with loci on 20q (EBN1) and 8q (EBN2). In contrast, the locus for Unverricht–Lundborg disease on chromosome 21q has been shown to also account for Mediterranean myoclonus. Two of the disease genes have been isolated by positional cloning: CLN1 and CLN3. The elucidation of ADNFLE nicely illustrates the power of present methodology. The region on 20q to which EBN1 maps was screened as a candidate region and linkage established. The transcript map in that region included a plausible candidate, CHRNA4, encoding the $\alpha 4$ subunit of the neuronal nicotinic acetylcholine receptor. Mutational analysis identified a base change causing an amino-acid substitution in a critical region which segregates with and clearly causes the disease (Steinlein *et al.*, 1995).

Application of linkage analysis to 'complex' familial epilepsies is much more problematic. If the phenotype arises from the interaction of several 'susceptibility loci' and environmental factors the relationship between genotype and phenotype is lost. Several complicating factors arise including the increased likelihood of genetic heterogeneity, low penetrance, difficulties in definition of the phenotype and uncertainty concerning the parameters of inheritance. Either parametric or 'nonparametric' methodology may be adopted, the latter including so-called affected sib-pair or affected pedigree member methods. The general effect is a loss of power, and large resources including several hundred sib-pairs may be necessary for success. The existence of high-resolution maps has made these diseases more tractable, and several loci for insulin-dependent diabetes mellitus (IDDM) have been identified.

Juvenile myoclonic epilepsy is the only common familial idiopathic generalized epilepsy which has been the subject of linkage studies. The mode of inheritance is 'complex' although studies have suggested autosomal-dominant, autosomal-recessive, two-locus and polygenic inheritance. Relatives of probands have an increased incidence of various idiopathic generalized epilepsy phenotypes and asymptomatic relatives may show a variety of electroencephalogram (EEG) abnormalities. Evidence in favour of a locus (EJM1) predisposing to JME in the HLA region of chromosome 6p was first obtained using serological markers (Greenberg et al., 1988). Linkage was subsequently replicated in a separately ascertained group of families (Weissbecker et al., 1991), and more recently evidence for a locus at a distance from HLA was obtained in a single large pedigree. However, further studies in a third set of families failed to find significant evidence in favour of linkage. These conflicting studies illustrate the difficulties inherent in applying linkage methodology to a trait which does not display Mendelian inheritance.

CANDIDATE GENE ANALYSIS

Analysis of candidate genes represents an alternative strategy, although there is clearly overlap as a candidate gene may be tested using linkage analysis. An obvious problem with this approach is the very high level and complexity of gene expression in neurones: in theory, any of the 30 000 different genes expressed in brain could be a candidate epilepsy gene.

The most plausible genes for involvement in the idiopathic epilepsies are those that play a direct role in mediating neuronal excitability in the central nervous system. These must include the genes encoding ion-channels, both voltage-gated and ligand-gated. In addition, the human homologues of murine epilepsy genes will represent candidate genes for human epilepsy (see below).

Mutations in ion-channels have now been shown to be responsible for a number of human diseases involving paroxysmal dysfunction of excitable tissues in brain, skeletal muscle and heart comparable to that which occurs in epilepsy. They can be divided into ligand-gated, e.g. the neurotransmitter receptors such as glutamate, GABA and acetylcholine receptors, and those that are voltage-gated, such as Na^+ and K^+ channels. Defects of inhibitory pathways (e.g. GABA-mediated Cl^- channels or K^+ channels) are perhaps an obvious, if simplistic, mechanism for generating excess excitability and seizures, but it is also easy to imagine situations in which mutations in genes mediating excitation may give rise to an epilepsy phenotype.

Most ion-channels are multimeric proteins and a very large number of genes, probably around one hundred or more, encoding subunits of these channels, have now been isolated and mapped in the human genome. For example, the functional $GABA_A$ receptor is a hetero-oligomeric structure the properties of which vary with subunit composition. At least four major subclasses of $GABA_A$ receptor subunit have been identified.

Analysis of candidate genes for epilepsy can be undertaken in one of two ways. First, linkage analysis as described above can be undertaken using a polymorphism that is either very close to or even within the gene of interest. This represents a more directed approach than that of a systematic genome search, but is still dependent on assumptions being made concerning the mode of inheritance and the penetrance of the disease-causing allele. Exclusion of a candidate gene can be established by demonstrating obligate recombination with an intragenic marker.

A second approach is direct mutational analysis of a candidate epilepsy gene. This approach involves amplification of the region of interest using the polymerase chain reaction in order to identify a variation affecting protein structure or expression. Mutation detection methods such as single strand conformation polymorphism (SSCP), heteroduplex analysis or direct DNA sequencing are applied to the polymerase chain reaction (PCR) product. This approach may be particularly valuable if there is significant genetic heterogeneity. It has been estimated that analysis of 50 affected individuals from different families would yield a 99% chance of identifying a mutation, even if only 10% of the families were linked to the gene under investigation.

Although the number of candidate epilepsy genes is large, the advent of automated sequencing and other time-saving methodologies makes the rapid mutational screening of a large number of genes possible in the near future.

MURINE MODELS

Models of epilepsy are well described in a number of species including chickens, primates and rodents (Buchhalter, 1993). Phenotypic and neurophysiological characterization is obviously easier in large animals, but for genetic analysis murine models are most favourable. There are several reasons for this. In particular, the mouse is a model organism for the human genome project and construction of genetic and physical maps of the mouse genome is well advanced. The mouse is easy to breed and suitable crosses for genetic mapping can easily be set up. Lastly, it is well established that a number of murine neurological disorders have exact homologies in man so identification of a mouse disease gene provides reasonable expectation that this will allow the corresponding human gene to be identified. These principles are illustrated by a description of the strategy being used to isolate the murine epilepsy gene, *lethargic*.

There are at least five single-locus recessive genetic disorders predisposing to generalized spike-wave epilepsy in the mouse. At present their molecular genetic basis is entirely unknown. Homozygous *lethargic (lh/lh)* mice develop spontaneous absence seizures at around 15 days of age. These seizures are accompanied by bilaterally synchronous bursts of 5–6 Hz spike-wave complexes, but there are no gross pathological changes in the central nervous system (CNS) or skeletal muscle.

The *lethargic* gene was originally mapped to mouse chromosome 2 by two-point linkage analysis with the Danforth's short tail locus (Sd) and found to lie between Sd and the agouti coat colour locus (a) in a region approximately 10–50 cM from the centromere. The following strategy is being adopted to achieve the isolation and characterization of the *lethargic* mouse epilepsy gene using positional cloning. The four major steps involved include: establishment of an interspecific backcross/intercross; high-resolution genetic mapping using polymorphic simple sequence repeats and identification of flanking markers; construction of a physical map across the region of interest; identification of genes within the region.

First, the mutant strain is crossed with another strain derived from an evolutionarily divergent mouse species or subspecies. This ensures that DNA markers which display variation between the two strains can be used to map accurately meiotic events and narrow down the disease gene region. A large interspecific cross has been established by crossing *lh/lh* homozygotes with several divergent but related species including M. m. castaneus. F_1 heterozygotes are then either mated together (intercross) or back to the original mutant strain (backcross).

DNA extracted from all F_2 and N_2 offspring is typed for a number of simple sequence length repeats along mouse chromosome 2. Haplotypes can then be built up and recombination breakpoints analysed to locate the mutant gene. Over 1000 meioses have now been analysed and flanking markers identified which are about 2 cM apart on mouse chromosome 2.

The next stage is to construct a physical map across this region. This is done by screening Yeast Artificial Chromosome (YAC), Bacterial Artificial Chromosome (BAC) and Pl (Phage) libraries to identify genomic clones from the critical region. Finally, gene isolation techniques such as exon trapping and direct cDNA selection will be used to construct a transcriptional map of the *lh* region. Genes within this region will be sequenced to identify the *lethargic* mutation.

The mouse *lh* cDNA will be used to screen a human brain cDNA library in order to identify the human homologue. This gene will represent a good candidate gene for human phenotypes such as childhood absence epilepsy.

In conclusion, powerful methods now exist for elucidating the molecular basis of human inherited epilepsies. The complex pattern of inheritance of common familial human epilepsies renders this a challenging task. An understanding of the pathophysiology of epilepsy at a molecular level will give rise to new methods for both diagnosis and treatment.

NOTE ADDED IN PROOF

The genes for two mouse models of epilepsy have now been cloned and shown to encode sub-units of voltage-dependant calcium channels. The *tottering* mouse is due to mutations in the α_{1A} gene (Fletcher *et al.*, 1996) and the *lethargic* mouse to mutations in *Cchb4* (Burgess *et al.*, 1997).

REFERENCES

Bird, T.D. (1992). Epilepsy. In: King, R.A., Rotter, J.I. and Motulsky, A.G. (Eds), *The Genetic Basis of Common Diseases, Vol. 20.* Oxford University Press, Oxford, pp. 732–752.

Buchhalter, J. (1993). Animal models of inherited epilepsy. *Epilepsia* **34** (suppl 3), 531–541.

Burgess, D.L., Jones, J.M., Meisler, M.H. and Noebels, J.L. (1997). Mutation of the Ca^{2+} channel β subunit gene *Cchb4* is associated with ataxia and seizures in the lethargic (*lh*) mouse. *Cell* **88**, 1–20.

Dichter, M.A. and Buchhalter, J.R. (1993). The genetic epilepsy. In: Rosenberg, R., Prusiner, S., Di Mauro, S., Barchi, R.L. and Kunkel, I.M. (Eds), *The Molecular and Genetic Basis of Neurological Disease.* Butterworth, Boston, MA, 925–947.

Fletcher, C.F., Lutz, C.M., O'Sullivan, T.N., Shaughnessy, Jr, J.D., Hawkes, R., Frankel, W.N., Copeland, N.G. and Jenkins, N.A. (1996). Absence epilepsy in tottering mice is associated with calcium channel defects. *Cell* **87**, 607–617.

Greenberg, D.A. Delgado-Escueta, A.V., Widelitz, H. *et al.* (1988). Juvenile myoclonic epilepsy may be linked to the BF and HLA loci on human chromosome 6. *Am J Med Genet* **31**, 185–192.

Lehesjoki, A.E., Koskiniemi, M., Sistonen, P. *et al.* (1991). Localisation of a gene for progressive myoclonus epilepsy to chromosome 21q22. *Proc Nat Acad Sci (USA)* **88**, 3696–3699.

Leppert, M., Anderson, V.E., Quattlebaum, T. *et al.* (1989). Benign familial neonatal convulsions linked to genetic markers on chromosome 20. *Nature* **337**, 647–648.

Leppert, M., McMahon, W., Quattlebaum, T. *et al.* (1993). Searching for human epilepsy genes: a progress report. *Brain Pathol* **3**, 357–369.

Lewis, T.B., Leach, R.J., Ward, K., O'Connell, P. and Ryan, S.G. (1993). Genetic heterogeneity in benign familial neonatal convulsions: identification of a new locus on chromosome 8q. *Am J Hum Genet* **53**, 670–675.

Ottman, R., Risch, N., Hauser, W.A. *et al.* (1995). Localization of a gene for partial epilepsy to chromosome 10q. *Nat Genet* **10**, 56–60.

Phillips, H.A., Scheffer, I.E., Bercovic, S.F., Hollway, G.E., Sutherland, G.R. and Mulley, J.C. (1995). Localization of a gene for autosomal dominant nocturnal frontal lobe epilepsy to Chromosome 20q13.2. *Nat Genet* **10**, 117–118.

Rees, M. and Gardiner, R. (1994). The epilepsies. In: Harding, A. (Ed.), *Genetics in Neurology, Vol. 3, No. 2.*, Baillière Tindall, London, pp. 297–313.

Serratosa, J.M., Delgado-Escueta, A.V., Posada, I. *et al.* (1995). The gene for progressive myoclonus epilepsy of the Lafora type maps to Chromosome 6q. *Hum Molec Genet* **5**, 1657–1663.

Steinlein, O.K., Mulley, J.C., Propping, P. *et al.* (1995). A missense mutation in the neuronal receptor α4 subunit is associated with autosomal dominant nocturnal frontal lobe epilepsy. *Nat Genet* **11**, 201–203.

Weissbecker, K.A., Durner, M., Janz, D., Scaramelli, A., Sparkes, R. and Spence, M. (1991). Confirmation of linkage between juvenile myoclonic epilepsy locus and the HLA region on chromosome 6. *Am J Med Genet* **38**, 32–36.

Epilepsy and Pregnancy
Edited by T. Tomson, L. Gram, M. Sillanpää and S.I. Johannessen
© 1997 Wrightson Biomedical Publishing Ltd

18

Localization of Epilepsy Genes – Where Are We Today?

ANNA-ELINA LEHESJOKI
Department of Medical Genetics, University of Helsinki, Finland

INTRODUCTION

Epilepsies are both clinically and aetiologically very heterogeneous (Commission on Classification and Terminology of the International League Against Epilepsy, 1989; Gardiner, 1990). A familial susceptibility to seizures has long been known and the genetics of various human epilepsies has been subject to numerous studies. In a minority of epilepsy patients, seizures occur as a component of a more complex phenotype displaying Mendelian inheritance; some 150 inherited disorders like this are known. In these disorders the effect on the neuronal function is often indirect and the underlying gene is not necessarily expressed in the brain (Gardiner, 1990). In 'pure' epilepsies, on the other hand, epileptic seizures occur as the sole or major symptom. Among these, one can distinguish a number of single-gene inherited disorders, but in all they are very rare. The inheritance pattern of the most common forms of epilepsies, showing familial clustering, does not conform to a simple Mendelian inheritance, and the inheritance pattern is usually concluded to be 'multifactorial', i.e. both genes and external factors are believed to contribute to the phenotype (Gardiner, 1990).

Linkage studies to localize epilepsy susceptibility genes have been performed in several epilepsy phenotypes. With one exception, at least one gene locus has been identified in each single-gene inherited epilepsy phenotype. However, in the multifactorial epilepsies linkage evidence (with highest logarithm-of-odds (lod) scores exceeding 3.0) on a susceptibility locus has been reported only in one phenotype: juvenile myoclonic epilepsy. Table 1 summarizes the epilepsy gene mapping data as of April 1996, and each individual phenotype is discussed in detail below.

Table 1. 'Pure' inherited forms of epilepsy, in which at least one gene locus has been identified.

Disease	Inheritance pattern[a]	Chromosomal localization[a]	Gene locus	Underlying gene
Juvenile myoclonic epilepsy	Multifactorial	?6p ?6p[b]	EJM1 EJM2	Not known Not known
Benign familial neonatal convulsions	AD	20q	EBN1	Not known
Benign familial neonatal convulsions	AD	8q[b]	EBN2	Not known
Nocturnal frontal lobe epilepsy	AD	20q[b]	CHRNA4	Alpha-4 neuronal nicotinic acetylcholine receptor subunit
Partial epilepsy	AD	10q[b]	EPT	Not known
Progressive myoclonus epilepsy of Unverricht–Lundborg type	AR	21q	CST6; EPM1	Cystatin B
Progressive epilepsy with mental retardation	AR	8p	EPMR	Not known

[a]p: short arm; q: long arm.
[b]Mapping evidence from a single large pedigree.
AD, autosomal dominant; AR, autosomal recessive.

JUVENILE MYOCLONIC EPILEPSY

Juvenile myoclonic epilepsy (JME) is a nonprogressive form of idiopathic generalized epilepsy (IGE). JME is estimated to account for 4–11% of all epilepsies (Delgado-Escueta et al., 1994). The key symptom is irregular bilateral myoclonic jerks, without loss of consciousness, which occur in otherwise healthy individuals (Asconape and Penry, 1984; Delgado-Escueta and Enrile-Bascal, 1984; Janz, 1985; Greenberg et al., 1988; Panayiotopoulos et al., 1989). The jerks occur mainly in the morning after awakening and can be provoked, for example, by lack of sleep. Myoclonic seizures are frequently accompanied by generalized tonic-clonic seizures, and in approximately 30% of the patients by absence seizures. In untreated patients the inter-ictal electroencephalogram (EEG) is typically abnormal, consisting of bilateral symmetrical diffuse 4–6 Hz multispike-and-wave complexes. Unaffected relatives may express similar EEG abnormalities (Tsuboi and Christian, 1973; Greenberg et al., 1988). Sodium valproate controls seizures in most JME patients. Family studies have demonstrated a clustering of JME or other IGEs in families with JME probands, but the underlying inheritance pattern remains uncertain, and several genetic factors are probably involved.

As JME displays a clear genetic basis, is relatively frequent and has a well defined phenotype it was identified almost 10 years ago as the most suitable of the non-Mendelian genetic epilepsies for linkage analysis. Greenberg *et al.* (1988) first reported positive linkage evidence to the HLA region in the short arm of chromosome 6 (6p) in families with probands with JME (gene locus designated EJM1). They studied 24 families and classified asymptomatic relatives with an abnormal EEG as affected. Linkage analysis using properdin factor B (BF) and HLA typing was carried out assuming either a fully penetrant recessive or a recessive with 60% penetrance inheritance model. When BF and HLA were analysed together, the lod score values were 3.04 (fully penetrant) and 3.03 (60% penetrance) (Greenberg *et al.*, 1988). The authors later presented additional evidence for linkage to BF and HLA and concluded that, whatever inheritance pattern is assumed, the lod score values stay over 3.0 as long as asymptomatic family members with an abnormal EEG are scored as affected (Greenberg *et al.*, 1989; Delgado-Escueta *et al.*, 1989). The group later reported that not all JME families are linked to EJM1 on chromosome 6p, suggesting genetic heterogeneity (Delgado-Escueta *et al.*, 1994; Liu *et al.*, 1995).

Weissbecker *et al.* (1991) studied 23 mostly nuclear families ascertained through a JME proband. Using HLA serologic markers they obtained the highest lod score value of 3.11 (at recombination fraction, θ, of 0.001 in males and 0.2 in females) assuming autosomal dominant inheritance with 90% penetrance. They classified asymptomatic individuals with an abnormal EEG as unaffected and included in the affected phenotype JME and other IGEs. The analysis of a subset of 20 of the 23 families, with extended family members and one new family, gave further evidence on EJM1 mapping close to the HLA region (Durner *et al.*, 1991). Sander *et al.* (1995) provided evidence that an IGE susceptibility gene maps to the HLA region and that the phenotypic spectrum includes JME, idiopathic absence epilepsies and epilepsies with generalized tonic-clonic seizures on awakening.

In a set of 25 families including a patient with JME and at least one first-degree relative with IGE, linkage analysis was carried out using eight polymorphic loci on chromosome 6p, and assuming autosomal-dominant and autosomal-recessive inheritance with age-dependent high or low penetrance (Whitehouse *et al.*, 1993). No significant evidence for linkage was obtained with any of the markers studied. The HLA region and a region 10–20 cM telomeric to HLA were excluded as a likely position of the EJM1 locus.

Recently, further evidence for a susceptibility locus for JME on 6p was obtained by the analysis of a single, large, four-generation pedigree with classical JME showing no pyknoleptic absences (Liu *et al.*, 1995). After a genome-wide search of 146 microsatellite polymorphisms, positive linkage evidence was obtained between the disease phenotype and chromosome 6p21.2-p11 markers, some 30 cM centromeric to the HLA region. The authors concluded that data from this large family independently proved that a JME gene, whose phenotype consists of classic JME with convulsions and/or EEG rapid multispike-and-wave complexes was located centromeric to HLA on chromosome 6p (Liu *et al.*, 1995).

Are there JME susceptibility loci on chromosome 6p? The data concerning EJM1 in the HLA region are still controversial. In the initial studies the highest lod scores were obtained after testing many different inheritance models and phenotype definitions, and therefore there is doubt about their exact statistical significance. Analysis of additional families has shown that not all families are linked to HLA, and genetic heterogeneity has been suggested to account for this. On the other hand, in an independent family set, no evidence for an EJM1 locus on 6p has been obtained. Clearly, further linkage studies under the assumption of genetic heterogeneity are needed to resolve these inconsistent findings. The mapping evidence for the JME locus centromeric to HLA derives from a single large pedigree. Analysis of additional pedigrees is needed to confirm this finding.

BENIGN FAMILIAL NEONATAL CONVULSIONS

Benign familial neonatal convulsions (BFNC) is a rare autosomal-dominant disorder (Zonana *et al.*, 1984). It is characterized by focal or generalized clonic seizures with onset typically during the first week of life and spontaneous remission by the age of six months (Rett and Teubel, 1964; Bjerre and Corelius, 1968; Dobrescu and Larbrisseau, 1982; Zonana *et al.*, 1984). Apart from seizures, no other signs of neuronal dysfunction are seen. Routine diagnostic studies are usually normal. Affected individuals almost invariably have normal growth and psychomotor development (Quattelbaum, 1979). In 10–20% of patients subsequent childhood or adult epilepsy develops, but the risk varies between families (Tibbles, 1980; Kaplan and Lacey, 1983; Zonana *et al.*, 1984; Shevell *et al.*, 1986; Ronen *et al.*, 1993).

BFNC was the first single-gene inherited epilepsy that was mapped to a specific genomic region. In 1989, Leppert and co-workers localized the BFNC gene, EBN1, to the long arm of chromosome 20 (20q) by linkage to DNA markers in a single, large, four-generation pedigree (Leppert *et al.*, 1989). Joint analysis of linkage between two marker loci, D20S19 and D20S20, and the disease phenotype gave a maximum lod score of 5.64 (θ = 0.00) (Leppert *et al.*, 1989). Subsequent analysis of additional families confirmed the existence of EBN1 on chromosome 20q (Ryan *et al.*, 1991; Malafosse *et al.*, 1992a; Berkovic *et al.*, 1994). Moreover, linkage evidence of heterogeneity was presented in one family in which the odds against linkage to EBN1 were greater than 20 000 : 1 (at $\theta \le 0.1$) (Ryan *et al.*, 1991).

As both clinical and linkage data suggested genetic heterogeneity, Lewis and co-workers started a random screen of the genome for linkage in one pedigree where linkage to chromosome 20q was excluded (Lewis *et al.*, 1993). After screening 21 markers, weak evidence for linkage to chromosome 8q was obtained. Analysis of additional markers proved linkage with a maximum pairwise lod score of 4.43 ($\theta = 0.00$) between the disease locus, EBN2, and markers D8S284 and D8S256 (Lewis *et al.*, 1993). The genetic length of the EBN2 region was estimated to be about 29 cM. In a second BFNC family, linkage to EBN1 was excluded and lod scores suggesting linkage (0.99 at D8S274) to EBN2 were detected (Steinlein *et al.*, 1995a). It was initially suggested that EBN1 would be associated with afebrile seizures beyond infancy, and that complete remission of BFNC would be specific to EBN2 (Lewis *et al.*, 1993; Berkovic *et al.*, 1994). However, three patients in a family with suggested linkage to 8q (Steinlein *et al.*, 1995a) showed subsequent epileptic seizures after 12 months of age.

BENIGN INFANTILE FAMILIAL CONVULSIONS

Benign infantile familial convulsions (BIFC) is a recently described benign epilepsy with an autosomal-dominant mode of inheritance (Vigevano *et al.*, 1992; Echenne *et al.*, 1994). The onset is between 3 and 12 months of age with clusters of partial seizures with secondary generalization (Vigevano *et al.*, 1992) or with clusters of brief generalized seizures (Echenne *et al.*, 1994). The seizures are well controlled by antiepileptic drugs and the outcome is favourable, with no recurrence of seizures after drug discontinuation. The inter-ictal EEG is usually normal as well as laboratory, radiological and neurological findings. By linkage analysis in eight BIFC families, using markers D20S19 and D20S20, a region of about 20 cM on each side of these markers was excluded as the location of the BIFC gene (Malafosse *et al.*, 1994). These data strongly suggest that EBN1 is not the gene implicated in BIFC.

AUTOSOMAL-DOMINANT NOCTURNAL FRONTAL LOBE EPILEPSY

Autosomal-dominant nocturnal frontal lobe epilepsy (ADNFLE) is the first reported partial epilepsy syndrome in humans that follows a single-gene inheritance (Scheffer *et al.*, 1994). The disorder is characterized by clusters of brief nocturnal motor seizures that almost exclusively occur during drowsing or sleep (Scheffer *et al.*, 1994, 1995). In milder cases the seizures are often misdiagnosed as nightmares or other sleep disorders. Onset is usually in childhood and seizures often persist throughout adult life. There is variable severity of symptoms in family members. Inter-ictal EEG is normal, but ictal recordings confirm that the attacks are partial seizures with frontal lobe seizure semiology (Scheffer *et al.*, 1994, 1995).

The underlying gene for ADNFLE has been assigned to chromosome 20q in the region where EBN1 resides in one Australian six-generation pedigree with 27 affected individuals (Phillips *et al.*, 1995). The highest lod score of 9.29 (θ = 0.00) was obtained at locus D20S19 (Phillips *et al.*, 1995). In the same family, Steinlein *et al.* (1995b) screened affected family members for mutations within an obvious candidate, the neuronal nicotinic acetylcholine receptor α4 subunit (CHRNA4) gene. The CHRNA4 gene had earlier been located in the ADNFLE region (Steinlein *et al.*, 1994) and was known to be expressed in all layers of the frontal cortex (Wevers *et al.*, 1994). A missense mutation, a C to T transition, was found to cosegregate with the disease phenotype in the family (Steinlein *et al.*, 1995b). The mutation replaces the neutral serine residue by the complex aromatic phenylalanine at codon 248, which is a strongly conserved amino acid residue in the second transmembrane domain of the protein. The mutation was present in all 21 available affected family members, but not in healthy control subjects. The mutation is expected to have a deleterious effect on the channel and is likely to be the disease-causing mutation (Steinlein *et al.*, 1995b). The authors reported that some other families with typical ADNFLE are not linked to chromosome 20q.

PARTIAL EPILEPSY

In an ongoing study of genetic contributions to epilepsy, Ottman and co-workers (1995) identified a single three-generation family with 11 affected individuals, in which an idiopathic/cryptogenic partial epilepsy phenotype segregated. The segregation pattern was compatible with autosomal-dominant inheritance showing a reduced penetrance. The age at onset of seizures was 8–19 years. In 10 out of the 11 affected individuals, the epilepsy was clearly localization-related. The remaining patient could not be classified because all seizures were nocturnal. Six patients had nonspecific auditory features as a simple partial component of the seizures (e.g. a ringing noise that grew louder). The inter-ictal EEG was normal. To localize the underlying gene, a random genome search was conducted. Positive linkage evidence was obtained on chromosome 10q, where a maximum pairwise lod score of 3.99 (θ = 0.00) was reached at marker D10S192 (Ottman *et al.*, 1995). All affected persons shared a seven-marker haplotype spanning 10 cM, and the maximum lod score for this haplotype was 4.83 (θ = 0.00). The data strongly suggested the existence of a gene, called EPT, affecting susceptibility to localization-related epilepsy on chromosome 10q.

PROGRESSIVE MYOCLONUS EPILEPSY OF UNVERRICHT–LUNDBORG TYPE

Progressive myoclonus epilepsy (PME) of Unverricht–Lundborg type, EPM1, is an autosomal-recessive disorder that has an incidence of at least

1 : 20 000 in Finland (Norio and Koskiniemi, 1979). It is relatively common also in the Mediterranean region (Malafosse *et al.*, 1992b; Lehesjoki *et al.*, 1994). The disorder is characterized by severe stimulus-sensitive myoclonus and tonic-clonic seizures (Koskiniemi *et al.*, 1974a; Norio and Koskiniemi, 1979; Koskiniemi, 1990). The age of onset is 6–15 years. The EEG findings are characteristic and sensitivity to photic stimulation is exceptionally high (Koskiniemi *et al.*, 1974b; Koskiniemi, 1990). Intellectual decline is slow. The seizures are usually well controlled by sodium valproate (Koskiniemi, 1990), but phenytoin is harmful (Eldridge *et al.*, 1983). Histopathologic examination reveals widespread degenerative changes but no evidence of storage material in the brain (Haltia *et al.*, 1969; Koskiniemi *et al.*, 1974a).

The EPM1 gene was assigned to chromosome 21q by linkage analysis in 12 Finnish families using polymorphic restriction fragment length (RFLP) markers (Lehesjoki *et al.*, 1991). Further genetic mapping in 13 multiplex families from Finland and one from the United States led to the assignment of EPM1 to an approximately 5 cM region between marker loci CBS and CD18 (Lehesjoki *et al.*, 1992, 1993a, b). By taking advantage of the unique features of the Finnish population (de la Chapelle, 1993), linkage disequilibrium was used to further narrow the localization of the EPM1 gene to a 0.6 cM or smaller region around loci D21S25, PFKL and D21S154 (Lehesjoki *et al.*, 1993b). The initial linkage disequilibrium data were mainly based on relatively poorly informative RFLP markers. Moreover, no polymorphic markers existed in an approximately 1 Mb region flanked by markers showing a high degree of linkage disequilibrium. Cloning of the region in bacterial clones (Stone *et al.*, 1996) allowed new markers to be identified and mapped. Subsequently, using haplotype analysis and historical recombination breakpoint mapping, with five highly polymorphic microsatellite markers covering some 900 kb of the EPM1 region, the gene was localized to a 175 kb region between marker loci D21S2040 and D21S1259 (Virtaneva *et al.*, 1996).

The localization of the EPM1 gene was precise enough to encourage the search for EPM1 candidate genes. The direct cDNA selection method was used to identify cDNA segments from the 175 kb region (Pennacchio *et al.*, 1996). Several of them encoded a previously described protein, cystatin B (CST6), a cysteine protease inhibitor (Järvinen and Rinne, 1982; Turk and Bode, 1991). Cystatin B is widely expressed and an mRNA approximately 0.8 kb in length is detected in Northern analysis. Analysis of lymphoblastoid cell mRNA showed that EPM1 patients had clearly reduced levels of cystatin B mRNA compared with non-carrier individuals and carrier parents (Pennacchio *et al.*, 1996). Sequence analysis of the cystatin B gene revealed two point mutations in affected individuals, a C to G transversion at the last nucleotide of intron 1, altering a splice site AG dinucleotide, and a C to T transition generating a translation stop codon at the amino acid position 68 (Pennacchio *et al.*, 1996). These changes were not present in unaffected individuals. The data provided evidence that mutations in the cystatin B gene are responsible for the primary defect in patients with EPM1.

Cystatin B is a 98 amino acid protein and member of a superfamily of cysteine protease inhibitors. It is a tightly binding reversible inhibitor of cathepsins L, J, S, and B (Järvinen and Rinne, 1982; Turk and Bode, 1991). It is found in all tissues and is thought to act as a protector against the proteinases leaking from lysosomes. It is not yet understood how mutations in the cystatin B cause the symptoms of EPM1.

PROGRESSIVE EPILEPSY WITH MENTAL RETARDATION

Progressive epilepsy with mental retardation (EPMR), or Northern epilepsy, is a new autosomal-recessively inherited disorder found recently in an isolated region in Finland where, with the exception of one, both parents of all of the 11 sibships with affected individuals descend from one or two founding couples (Hirvasniemi et al., 1994). EPMR is characterized by normal early development, the onset of generalized tonic-clonic seizures at 5–10 years and progressive mental retardation beginning two to five years after the first seizures (Hirvasniemi et al., 1994, 1995). The seizures increase in frequency, reaching approximately 4–10 seizures per month during puberty, after which the frequency of seizures diminishes. After 35 years of age, many patients are virtually seizure-free. Mental deterioration is rapid in the early stage of the disease and by the age of 30 years all patients show an IQ of less than 70; by 40 years all are at least moderately retarded (Hirvasniemi et al., 1995). Clonazepam appears to be the most effective antiepileptic drug in EPMR. EEG shows progressive slowing of background activity until puberty, after which the delta and theta activity diminishes and slow alpha activity reappears (Hirvasniemi et al., 1994). Epileptiform activity is scarce during all stages of the disease. In computerized tomography (CT) scans progressive cerebellar-brainstem and cerebral atrophy is seen (Hirvasniemi and Karumo, 1994). Routine laboratory test findings are usually normal (Hirvasniemi et al., 1994).

As the biochemical defect underlying EPMR was not known, a random search of the genome was performed to localize the EPMR gene. After testing 153 microsatellite markers, linkage was observed with marker D8S264 on chromosome 8p (Tahvanainen et al., 1994). Linkage was confirmed with four additional markers. The EPMR gene was found to reside in an approximately 7 cM interval between marker loci D8S262 on the centromeric and AFM185xb2 on the telomeric side, where a maximum multipoint lod score of 7.03 was obtained 1.8 cM centromeric to D8S264. Haplotype analysis supported the hypothesis of a single founding mutation for all affected chromosomes, except the one belonging to the unrelated parent, who had a very different haplotype. This finding suggests the existence of another mutation or a very old ancestry of a single mutation.

By analysing new markers from the EPMR gene region, the gene localization has further been narrowed to some 4 cM (Ranta *et al.*, 1996). A yeast artificial chromosome (YAC) contig containing 22 YACs and covering a minimum of 3 Mb, has been constructed across the disease gene region. New polymorphic markers have been identified from the region and are being analysed to narrow the region further by refining the recombination breakpoints and by haplotype analysis. Attempts to clone candidate genes from the region are under way.

CONCLUSION

Gene localization has been relatively straightforward in the two 'Finnish' autosomal recessive epilepsies that are clinically and genetically quite homogeneous. Experience from two single-gene inherited, autosomal dominant epilepsies, BFNC and ADNFLE, on the other hand, indicates that these disorders are heterogeneous, both concerning phenotype and the genetic background. This implies that the phenotype-to-genotype relationship can be even more complex in multifactorial epilepsies. This has actually been shown to be the case in juvenile myoclonic epilepsy, in which data obtained from different studies are inconsistent. It has been proposed (Berkovic *et al.*, 1994) that studying single large multiplex families in which problems of genotypic heterogeneity are likely to be minimized may be the best approach to identifying susceptibility genes in the more common forms of epilepsy. Alternatively, analysis of a large set of multiple small families under the assumption of genetic heterogeneity is needed. Attempts to collect such family panels with various epilepsy phenotypes are ongoing.

REFERENCES

Asconape, J. and Penry, J.K. (1984). Some clinical and EEG aspects of benign juvenile myoclonic epilepsy. *Epilepsia* **25**, 108–114.

Berkovic, S.F., Kennerson, M.L., Howell, R.A., Scheffer, I.E., Hwang, P.A. and Nicholson, G.A. (1994). Phenotypic expression of benign familial neonatal convulsions linked to chromosome 20. *Arch Neurol* **51**, 1125–1128.

Bjerre, I. and Corelius, E. (1968). Benign familial neonatal convulsions. *Acta Paediatr Scand* **57**, 557–561.

Commission on Classification and Terminology of the International League Against Epilepsy (1989). Proposal for revised classification of epilepsies and epileptic syndromes. *Epilepsia* **30**, 389–399.

de la Chapelle, A. (1993). Disease gene mapping in isolated human populations: the example of Finland. *J Med Genet* **30**, 857–865.

Delgado-Escueta, A.V. and Enrile-Bascal, F.E. (1984). Juvenile myoclonic epilepsy of Janz. *Neurology* **34**, 285–294.

Delgado-Escueta, A.V., Greenberg, D.A., Treiman, L. *et al.* (1989). Mapping the gene for juvenile myoclonic epilepsy. *Epilepsia* **30** (suppl 4), 8–18.

Delgado-Escueta, A.V., Serratosa, J.M., Liu, A.*et al.* (1994). Progress in mapping human epilepsy genes. *Epilepsia* **35** (suppl 1), 29–40.

Dobrescu, O. and Larbrisseau, A. (1982). Benign familial neonatal convulsions. *Can J Neurol Sci* **9**, 345–347.

Durner, M., Sander, T., Greenberg, D.A., Johnson, K., Beck-Mannagetta, G. and Janz, D. (1991). Localization of idiopathic generalized epilepsy on chromosome 6p in families of juvenile myoclonic epilepsy patients. *Neurology* **41**, 1651–1655.

Echenne, B., Humbertclaude, V., Rivier, F., Malafosse, A. and Cheminal, R. (1994). Benign infantile epilepsy with autosomal dominant inheritance. *Brain Dev* **16**, 108–111.

Eldridge, R., Livanainen, M., Stern, R., Koerber, T. and Wilder, B.J. (1983). 'Baltic' myoclonus epilepsy: hereditary disorder of childhood made worse by phenytoin. *Lancet* **ii**, 838–842.

Gardiner, R.M. (1990). Genes and epilepsy. *J Med Genet* **27**, 537–544.

Greenberg, D.A., Delgado-Escueta, A.V., Widelitz, H. *et al.*, (1988). Juvenile myoclonic epilepsy (JME) may be linked to the BF and HLA lock on human chromosome 6. *Am J Med Genet* **31**, 185–192.

Greenberg, D.A., Delgado-Escueta, A.V., Widelitz, H., Abad, P. and Park, M.S. (1989). Strengthened evidence for linkage of juvenile myoclonic epilepsy to HLA and BF (Abstract). *Cytogenet Cell Genet* **51**, 1008.

Haltia, M., Kristensson, K. and Sourander, P. (1969). Neuropathological studies in three Scandinavian cases of progressive myoclonus epilepsy. *Acta Neurol Scand* **45**, 63–77.

Hirvasniemi, A. and Karumo, J. (1994). Neuroradiological findings in the Northern epilepsy syndrome. *Acta Neurol Scand* **90**, 388–393.

Hirvasniemi, A., Lang, H., Lehesjoki, A.-E. and Leisti, J. (1994). Northern epilepsy syndrome: an inherited childhood onset epilepsy with associated mental deterioration. *J Med Genet* **31**, 177–182.

Hirvasniemi, A., Herrala, P. and Leisti, J. (1995). Northern epilepsy syndrome: clinical course and the effect of medication on seizures. *Epilepsia* **36**, 792–797.

Janz, D. (1985). Epilepsy with impulsive petit mal (juvenile myoclonic epilepsy). *Acta Neurol Scand* **72**, 449–459.

Järvinen, M. and Rinne, A. (1982). Human spleen cysteine proteinase inhibitor: purification, fractionation into isoelectric variants and some properties of the variants. *Biochim Biophys Acta* **707**, 210–217.

Kaplan, R.E. and Lacey, D.J. (1983). Benign familial neonatal-infantile seizures. *Am J Med Genet* **16**, 595–599.

Koskiniemi, M. (1990). Progressive myoclonic epilepsy. In: Sillanpää, M., Johannessen, S.I., Blennow, G. and Dam, M. (Eds), *Paediatric Epilepsy*. Wrightson Biomedical, Petersfield, Hampshire, pp. 137–144.

Koskiniemi, M., Donner, M., Majuri, H., Haltia, M. and Norio, R. (1974a). Progressive myoclonus epilepsy: a clinical and histopathological study. *Acta Neurol Scand* **50**, 307–322.

Koskiniemi, M., Toivakka, E. and Donner, M. (1974b). Progressive myoclonus epilepsy. Electroencephalographical findings. *Acta Neurol Scand* **50**, 333–359.

Lehesjoki, A.-E., Koskiniemi, M., Sistonen, P. *et al.* (1991). Localization of a gene for progressive myoclonus epilepsy to chromosome 21q22. *Proc Natl Acad Sci* **88**, 3696–3699.

Lehesjoki, A.-E., Koskiniemi, M., Pandolfo, M. *et al.* (1992). Linkage studies in progressive myoclonus epilepsy: Unverricht–Lundborg and Lafora's diseases. *Neurology* **42**, 1545–1550.

Lehesjoki, A.-E., Eldridge, R., Eldridge, J., Wilder, B.J. and de la Chapelle, A. (1993a). Progressive myoclonus epilepsy of Unverricht–Lundborg type: a clinical and molecular genetic study of a family from the United States with four affected sibs. *Neurology* **43**, 2384–2386.

Lehesjoki, A.-E., Koskiniemi, M., Norio, R. *et al.* (1993b). Localization of the EPM1 gene for progressive myoclonus epilepsy on chromosome 21: linkage disequilibrium allows high-resolution mapping. *Hum Molec Genet* **2**, 1229–1234.

Lehesjoki, A.-E., Tassinari, C.A., Avanzini, G. *et al.* (1994). PME of Unverricht–Lundborg type in the Mediterranean region: linkage and linkage disequilibrium confirm the assignment to the EPM1 locus. *Hum Genet* **93**, 668–674.

Leppert, M., Anderson, V.E., Quattlebaum, T. *et al.* (1989). Benign familial neonatal convulsions linked to genetic markers on chromosome 20. *Nature* **337**, 647–648.

Lewis, T.B., Leach, R.J., Ward, K., O'Connell, P. and Ryan, S.G. (1993). Genetic heterogeneity in benign familial neonatal convulsions: identification of a new locus on chromosome 8q. *Am J Hum Genet* **53**, 670–675.

Liu, A.W., Delgado-Escueta, A.V., Serratosa, J.M. *et al.* (1995). Juvenile myoclonic epilepsy locus in chromosome 6p21.2-p11: linkage to convulsions and electroencephalography trait. *Am J Hum Genet* **57**, 368–381.

Malafosse, A., Leboyer, M., Dulac, O. *et al.* (1992a). Confirmation of linkage of benign familial neonatal convulsions to D20S19 and D20S20. *Hum Genet* **89**, 54–58.

Malafosse, A., Lehesjoki, A.-E., Genton, P. *et al.* (1992b). Identical genetic locus for Baltic and Mediterranean myoclonus. *Lancet* **339**, 1080–1081.

Malafosse, A., Beck, C., Bellet, H. *et al.* (1994). Benign infantile familial convulsions are not an allelic form of the benign familial neonatal convulsions gene. *Ann Neurol* **35**, 479–482.

Norio, R. and Koskiniemi, M. (1979). Progressive myoclonus epilepsy: genetic and nosological aspects with special reference to 107 Finnish patients. *Clin Genet* **15**, 382–398.

Ottman, R., Risch, N., Hauser, W.A. *et al.* (1995). Localization of a gene for partial epilepsy to chromosome 10q. *Nat Genet* **10**, 56–60.

Panayiotopoulos, C.P., Obeid, T. and Waheed, G. (1989). Absences in juvenile myoclonic epilepsy: a clinical and video-electroencephalographic study. *Ann Neurol* **25**, 391–397.

Pennacchio, L.A., Lehesjoki, A.-E., Stone, N.E. *et al.* (1996). Mutations in the gene encoding cystatin B in progressive myoclonus epilepsy (EPM1). *Science* **271**, 1731–1734.

Phillips, H.A., Scheffer, I.E., Berkovic, S.F., Hollway, G.E., Sutherland, G.R. and Mulley, J.C. (1995). Localization of a gene for autosomal dominant nocturnal frontal lobe epilepsy to chromosome 20q13.2. *Nat Genet* **10**, 117–118.

Quattlebaum, T.G. (1979). Benign familial neonatal convulsions in the neonatal period and early infancy. *J Pediatr* **95**, 257–259.

Ranta, S., Lehesjoki, A.E., Hirvasniemi, A. *et al.* (1996). Genetic and physical mapping of the progressive epilepsy with mental retardation (EPMR) locus on chromosome 8p. *Genome Res* **6**, 351–360.

Rett, A. and Teubel, R. (1964). Neugeborenenkraempfe in Rahmen einer epileptisch belasteten Familie. *Wien Klin Wochenschr* **76**, 609–613.

Ronen, G.M., Rosales, T.O., Connolly, M., Anderson, V.E. and Leppert, M. (1993). Seizure characteristics in chromosome 20 benign familial neonatal convulsions. *Neurology* **43**, 1355–1360.

Ryan, S.G., Wiznitzer, M., Hollman, C., Torres, M.C., Szekeresova, M. and Schneider, S. (1991). Benign familial neonatal convulsions: evidence for clinical and genetic heterogeneity. *Ann Neurol* **29**, 469–473.

Sander, T., Hildman, T., Janz, D. *et al.* (1995). The phenotypic spectrum related to the human epilepsy susceptibility gene 'EJM1'. *Ann Neurol* **38**, 210–217.

Scheffer, I.E., Bhatia, K.P., Lopes-Cendes, I. *et al.* (1994). Autosomal dominant frontal epilepsy misdiagnosed as sleep disorder. *Lancet* **343**, 515–517.

Scheffer, I.E., Bhatia, K.P., Lopes-Cendes, I. *et al.* (1995). Autosomal dominant nocturnal frontal epilepsy: a distinctive clinical disorder. *Brain* **118**, 61–73.

Shevell, M.I., Sinclair, D.B. and Metrakos, K. (1986). Benign familial neonatal seizures: clinical and electroencephalographic characteristics. *Pediatr Neurol* **2**, 272–275.

Steinlein, O., Smigrodzki, R., Lindstrom, J. *et al.* (1994). Refinement of the localization of the gene for neuronal nicotinic acetylcholine receptor alpha-4 subunit (CHRNA4) to human chromosome 20q13.2-q13.3. *Genomics* **22**, 493–495.

Steinlein, O., Schuster, V., Fischer, C. and Haussler, M. (1995a). Benign familial neonatal convulsions: confirmation of genetic heterogeneity and further evidence for a second locus on chromosome 8q. *Hum Genet* **95**, 411–415.

Steinlein, O.K., Mulley, J.C., Propping, P. *et al.* (1995b). A misssense mutation in the neuronal nicotinic acetylcholine receptor alpha-4 subunit is associated with autosomal dominant nocturnal frontal lobe epilepsy. *Nat Genet* **11**, 201–203.

Stone, N.E., Fan, J.-B., Willour, V. *et al.* (1996). Construction of a 750 kb bacterial clone contig and restriction map in the region of human chromosome 21 containing the progressive myoclonus epilepsy (EPM1) gene. *Genome Res* **6**, 218–225.

Tahvanainen, E., Ranta, S., Hirvasniemi, A. *et al.* (1994). The gene for a recessively inherited human childhood progressive epilepsy with mental retardation maps to the distal short arm of chromosome 8. *Proc Natl Acad Sci* **91**, 7267–7270.

Tibbles, J.A.R. (1980). Dominant benign neonatal seizures. *Dev Med Child Neurol* **22**, 664–667.

Tsuboi, T. and Christian, W. (1973). On the genetics of primary generalized epilepsy with sporadic myoclonias of impulsive petit mal type. *Humangenetik* **19**, 155–182.

Turk, V. and Bode, W. (1991). The cystatins: protein inhibitors of cysteine proteinases. *FEBS Lett* **285**, 213–219.

Vigevano, F., Fusco, L., Di Capua, M., Ricci, S., Sebastianelli, R. and Lucchini, P. (1992). Benign infantile familial convulsions. *Eur J Pediatr* **151**, 608–612.

Virtaneva, K., Miao, J., Träskelin, A.-L. *et al.* (1996). Progressive myoclonus epilepsy EPM1 locus maps to a 175 kb interval in distal 21q. *Am J Hum Genet* 1997 (in press).

Weissbecker, K.A., Durner, M., Janz, D., Scaramelli, A., Sparkes, R.S. and Spence, M.A. (1991). Confirmation of linkage between juvenile myoclonic epilepsy locus and the HLA region of chromosome 6. *Am J Med Genet* **38**, 32–36.

Wevers, A., Jeske, A., Lobron, C. *et al.* (1994). Cellular distribution of nicotinic acetylcholine receptor subunit mRNAs in the human cerebral cortex as revealed by non-isotopic *in situ* hybridization. *Brain Res Mol Brain Res* **25**, 122–128.

Whitehouse, W.P., Rees, M., Curtis, D. *et al.* (1993). Linkage analysis of idiopathic generalized epilepsy (IGE) and marker loci on chromosome 6p in families of patients with juvenile myoclonic epilepsy: no evidence for an epilepsy locus in the HLA region. *Am J Hum Genet* **53**, 652–662.

Zonana, J., Silvey, K. and Strimling, B. (1984). Familial neonatal and infantile seizures: an autosomal-dominant disorder. *Am J Med Genet* **18**, 455–459.

Epilepsy and Pregnancy
Edited by T. Tomson, L. Gram, M. Sillanpää and S.I. Johannessen
© 1997 Wrightson Biomedical Publishing Ltd

19

What is the Risk of Inheriting Epilepsy?

MATTI SILLANPÄÄ

Department of Child Neurology, University of Turku, Turku, Finland

INTRODUCTION

Questions about inheritance are more and more often asked by patients with epilepsy. This is in part a consequence of progress made in molecular genetics and new information given by researchers. Undoubtedly, genetics plays a remarkable role in epilepsy. Increasing knowledge of the inheritance of epilepsy warrants improved genetic counselling, not least in prepregnancy situations. Although every epilepsy is not necessarily inherited, genetic factors must be considered in every patient suffering from epileptic seizures. The manifestation and phenotype of epilepsy are influenced by heritability, penetrance and expressivity.

Heritability of liability to epilepsy, i.e. the proportion of total variance explained by genetic factors, generally varies from one pattern of inheritance to another: in autosomal-dominant pattern, 50%, in autosomal-recessive, 25% equally in males and females, and X-linked recessive in 50% of males. Population-based twin studies suggest that 8–27% of the incidence of epileptic seizures is related to genetic variability (Sillanpää *et al.*, 1991). Penetrance, i.e. the proportion of carriers who show any clinical expression (phenotype) of the disease, may be complete or incomplete. The incompleteness of penetrance may result from early death before reaching the age of onset and therefore skipping one pedigree, from low expressivity (failure to detect minimal signs), or from genetic or environmental factors modifying the penetrance.

Risk is a probability that an untoward event will occur. It is a theoretical concept and refers to individuals (Miettinen, 1985). As we know, it is difficult to predict the future. It is no less difficult to predict the risk of future epilepsy appearing in an individual. In the evaluation of the risk of inheriting epilepsy, the patterns of inheritance of different epilepsies should be known in order to enable genetic evaluation of patients with epilepsy. Modes

Table 1. Mendelian traits associated with seizures.

Mode of inheritance	Total (n)	With seizures	
		n	%
Autosomal-dominant	3 047	46	1.4
Autosomal-recessive	1 554	98	6.3
X-linked	336	19	5.7
Total	4 937	160	3.2

Source: McKusick, 1990.

of inheritance of epilepsy may be monogenic (Mendelian), heterogenic (polygenic, multifactorial), mitochondrial, and nongenetic.

MENDELIAN INHERITANCE

More than 150 of approximately 5000 diseases with Mendelian inheritance (McKusick, 1990) show an increased risk of epilepsy (Table 1). The possibility of Mendelian inheritance must always be considered if there are several family members or first-degree relatives with epilepsy. This is despite the fact that Mendelian inherited epilepsies account for only 1–2% of the epileptic population.

Autosomal-dominant inheritance

In general, in diseases with autosomal-dominant inheritance only one defective allele locus is needed to manifest the disease and penetrance is incomplete. Autosomal-dominantly inherited diseases are relatively easy to detect because 50% of people with an autosomal-dominant gene are affected, the disorder is then rather common, and occurs in several successive generations. Males and females are equally affected, there is male-to-male transmission, and affected people occur in multiple generations with highly variable expression. The diseases are often less severe, the survival rate is high, and seizures are less common (Table 2). Abnormal cell surface activity or structural proteins are mostly responsible for the occurrence of the disease.

Ninety percent of patients with tuberous sclerosis have epileptic seizures. Inheritance is characterized by a reduced penetrance and a high mutation rate. Linkage studies have identified several gene loci for tuberous sclerosis.

Neurofibromatosis type I or von Recklinghausen's disease is an autosomal-dominantly inherited disorder with the incidence of 1 : 3000. Epilepsy occurs in about 30% of people with neurofibromatosis type I but is usually not a presenting symptom. This disorder is characterized by a high mutation rate and often unique mutations.

Table 2. Examples of autosomal-
dominant epilepsies.

Tuberous sclerosis
Neurofibromatosis type I
Huntington's disease
Benign familial neonatal convulsions
Nocturnal frontal lobe epilepsy
Partial epilepsy with auditory symptoms

Huntington's disease usually has its onset in adulthood but in 5–10% of cases onset occurs in childhood. Generalized tonic-clonic, myoclonic and atypical absence seizures are relatively common in childhood-onset disease compared with adults whose incidence of seizures is about 10%.

Benign familial neonatal convulsions was the first epileptic syndrome where linkage analysis was successfully used to determine the gene locus. A 41% incidence in at-risk infants with no sex-linked transmission argues for an autosomal-dominant inheritance with high but not complete penetrance (Zonana *et al.*, 1984). A gene for autosomal-dominant nocturnal frontal lobe epilepsy has been mapped to the same chromosome, 20q, as benign familial neonatal convulsions, suggesting a situation of allelic variants (Phillips *et al.*, 1995). In addition to incomplete penetrance, an intrafamilial variability in severity from nightmares to frequent nocturnal convulsions exists (Scheffer *et al.*, 1994).

A partial epilepsy with frequent auditory symptoms and with a strong evidence of autosomal dominant inheritance has recently been reported (Ottman *et al.*, 1995b).

Autosomal-recessive inheritance

An autosomal-recessive disorder is clinically manifested when both alleles at a locus are defective and both parents are then heterogenous carriers for the disease. Hence, offspring with heterogenous parents have a 25% risk of being homozygous and having the disease. Typically, one generation only is affected. These diseases are often rare but, if consanguinity is found, an autosomal-recessive inheritance should be considered. In this type of inheritance, there is often an enzyme defect typically resulting in early onset, high frequency of seizures and mental retardation, and severe course of the disease (Table 3).

Progressive myoclonus epilepsy of the Unverricht–Lundborg type, the Mediterranean type, and Baltic type seem homologous. Consanguinity rate is high, and the proportion of affected siblings is 26%, appropriate to autosomal-recessive inheritance (Norio and Koskiniemi, 1979).

Neuronal ceroid lipofuscinosis consists of several subforms: infantile, late infantile, late infantile variant, juvenile, and adult Kufs type. Epilepsy occurs

Table 3. Examples of autosomal-
recessive epilepsies.

Progressive myoclonus epilepsy
Juvenile neuronal ceroid lipofuscinosis
Infantile neuronal ceroid lipofuscinosis
Progressive encephalopathy with oedema,
hypsarrhythmia and optic atrophy
Northern epilepsy

especially in juvenile type but also in infantile types. Age at onset of seizures is associated with the onset of the disease.

Progressive encephalopathy with oedema, hypsarrhythmia and optic atrophy or the PEHO syndrome is an apparently autosomal-recessive disorder with a rare familial occurrence of infantile spasms (Salonen *et al.*, 1991). Its minimum estimated incidence in Finland is 1 : 74 000. The same syndrome has been suspected but not proved in the UK, Sweden, France and Japan. After infantile spasms, almost all patients continued to have drug-resistant seizures reminiscent of those found in the Lennox–Gastaut syndrome (Somer, 1993).

Northern epilepsy is one of the newest autosomal-recessively inherited types of epilepsy belonging to the Finnish disease heritage (Hirvasniemi *et al.*, 1994). As yet identified only in a small area of the north-eastern part of Finland, it has been demonstrated to occur consanguineously in nine families, with a common ancestor having been traced back to the first half of the seventeenth century. The gene has been localized to chromosome 8p (Tahvanainen *et al.*, 1994). The typical age at onset of epilepsy is 5–10 years, with the frequency of seizures decreasing in young adulthood (Hirvasniemi *et al.*, 1994).

X-linked inheritance

In X-linked recessive inheritance males are largely affected because of a good expressivity of the single X chromosome of males but poor expressivity of the females who are most likely heterogenous and therefore carriers for that disease. A disorder which occurs in males only is usually easy to detect if the disorder has been characteristically transmitted through unaffected females. In genetic counselling, both the limiting effect of the carrier state on reproduction and the possibility of a new mutation must be taken into account (Table 4).

Menkes' kinky hair disease was identified as an X-linked disease in 1962 and as resulting from a defect in copper metabolism in 1972. Seizures occur in all patients and have their onset by the age of three months, accompanied by developmental delay and early death (Holmes, 1987). Lesch–Nyhan

Table 4. Examples of X-linked epilepsies.

Fragile-X syndrome
Menkes' kinky hair disease
Lesch–Nyhan disease
Pelizaeus–Merzbacher disease

disease, a disorder of uric acid metabolism, has its onset at the age of about three months. Motor and mental deterioration during the first year of life, self-mutilation behaviour and uric acid crystalluria in a male infant are suggestive of the disease which may be confirmed by identifying a specific enzyme defect. Seizures occur in 50% of patients. In 15% of classic and adult forms of Pelizaeus–Merzbacher disease, a sudanophilic leucodystrophy, epilepsy is accompanied by other neurological symptoms.

Chromosomal abnormalities

Several common chromosomal abnormalities present with epileptic seizures. In Down's syndrome, an increase in the incidence of seizures may be seen in advancing age and particularly in association with the occurrence of Alzheimer-like histological changes in the brain (Sim *et al.*, 1966). The incidence of epilepsy in patients with Alzheimer's disease but without Down's syndrome is 10% (Hauser *et al.*, 1986) but in patients with Down's syndrome and Alzheimer-like dementia 75% or more (Lai and Williams, 1989), a fact that refers to a specific epileptogenic factor in Down's patients (Stafstrom, 1993). The fragile-X syndrome, a rival to Down's syndrome as a specific cause of mental retardation, may be associated with epileptic seizures in 24–42% of patients (Musumeci *et al.*, 1988). An EEG pattern may be reminiscent of those in benign rolandic epilepsy, but any type of seizure may occur. In mental retardation, the chromosomal analysis is of the utmost importance in detecting the fragile-X or other chromosomal abnormalities. Epilepsy is common in patients with a ring chromosome 20 (Back *et al.*, 1989; Holopainen *et al.*, 1994). A small deletion of chromosome 15, inherited from the maternal side, results in Angelman syndrome but, inherited from paternal side, causes Prader–Willi syndrome. Seizures are common in Angelman syndrome but infrequent in Prader–Willi syndrome.

Mitochondrial inheritance

At least two maternally transmitted disorders with a mutation in the mitochondrial genome and defective mitochondrial energy production are known to date. In mitochondrial inheritance all children are at risk, but the disorder is highly variable in expression and severity. Variations include

Table 5. Mitochondrially inherited epilepsies.

Myoclonic epilepsy with ragged red fibres
Mitochondrial encephalopathy, lactic acidosis, and
stroke-like episodes
Infantile-onset myoclonic epilepsy

myoclonic epilepsy with ragged red fibres (MERRF) and mitochondrial encephalopathy, lactic acidosis and stroke-like episodes (MELAS). In addition, an infantile-onset progressive myoclonic epilepsy has been identified (Table 5).

MERRF has its onset between 5 and 15 years and includes muscle weakness, intention myoclonus, progressive ataxia, deafness and epilepsy. Several members of one family with different ages may have various types of seizures. Epilepsy is included by definition in MERRF but is also very common in MELAS, comprising 94% of all patients with that disorder in one series (DiMauro *et al.*, 1991). In MELAS, focal seizures and even epilepsia partialis continua are relatively common (Montagna *et al.*, 1988). An infantile-onset progressive myoclonus epilepsy presents with myoclonic seizures, generalized tonic-clonic seizures and neurodevelopmental delay or regression, and bilateral multifocal paroxysmal discharges in a slow background activity (Harbord *et al.*, 1991).

HETEROGENIC (NON-MENDELIAN) INHERITANCE

While Mendelian inheritance is estimated to account for no more than 1–2% of the population with epilepsy, the vast majority have a more complex genetics of epilepsy with a substantially lower risk of epilepsy than in a single-locus Mendelian inheritance. Multifactorial inheritance is a mixture of genetic and environmental aetiological factors. This combination may be expected in families where there is an overrepresentation of epilepsy but no evidence of a Mendelian inheritance or chromosomal abnormality. In three common familial epilepsy syndromes, genetic factors have been strongly suggested to be contributary to the aetiology. These are juvenile myoclonic epilepsy, childhood absence epilepsy, and benign rolandic epilepsy.

Juvenile myoclonic epilepsy

Juvenile myoclonic epilepsy comprises 5–10% of all epilepsies. It is characterized by myoclonic jerks on awakening, generalized tonic-clonic convulsions and typical daytime pyknoleptic seizures. The gene defect has been localized in the short arm of chromosome 6 (Greenberg *et al.*, 1988).

However, the mode of inheritance is not clear. Evidence for several patterns of inheritance has been obtained, including autosomal-dominant (Delgado-Escueta *et al.*, 1990), autosomal-recessive (Panayiotopoulos and Obeid, 1989), two-locus (Greenberg *et al.*, 1989), and multifactorial (Andermann, 1982). The conflicting results could be explained by a gene locus heterogeneity.

Childhood absence epilepsy

Childhood absence epilepsy occurs in 8% of school-age children, with the majority (60–75%) in girls. A positive family history has been reported in 15–44% (Currier *et al.*, 1963; Lugaresi *et al.*, 1973). In twins, the concordance rate for absence epilepsy is 75% and for 3 Hz spike-wave electroencephalogram (EEG) 84% (Lennox, 1951). The pattern of inheritance is unclear; evidence for autosomal-dominant (Metrakos and Metrakos, 1972) and for autosomal-recessive inheritance (Serratosa *et al.*, 1990) exists.

Benign rolandic epilepsy

Benign rolandic epilepsy has its onset between 5 and 10 years, with typically orofacial seizures occurring on awakening or soon thereafter. A positive family history of seizures is reportedly up to 68% with typical centrotemporal spike foci in 30% (Gardiner, 1996). The EEG findings have been suggested to be inherited autosomal-dominantly with an age-dependent penetrance (Bray and Wiser, 1965; Heijbel *et al.*, 1975).

Epilepsy with grand mal upon awakening

Juvenile myoclonic epilepsy as well as the adolescence-onset form of primary idiopathic generalized epilepsy have a gene locus on chromosome 6. However, not all adolescence-onset idiopathic generalized epilepsies appear to be on that gene locus. In all probability there are clinically similar epileptic syndromes with different genetic grounds. Therefore, it is of the utmost importance to collect precise and reliable clinical data for the basis of seizure and epilepsy diagnosis (Greenberg *et al.*, 1995).

NONGENETIC AETIOLOGY

In clinical practice the vast majority of patients have no identified genetic basis for epilepsy. Reasons for a negative family history of epilepsy may be, for example, unidentified epilepsy, identified acquired epilepsy, recall bias in case of an age-dependent expressivity, or death before onset of epilepsy. The patient may have a new mutation, or may have an acquired cause of epilepsy. The mutation may be (almost solely) responsible for epilepsy, a coincidental event, or 'antecedent' to epilepsy (Anderson and Hauser, 1991). The family history is positive for epilepsy more frequently in patients who have seizures in association with brain tumour, or in spastic hemiplegia (7% versus 2%). Except for a few known gene defects, most epilepsies with onset before the age of six months are likely to have a nongenetic aetiology (Hauser and Annegers, 1991).

EVALUATION OF RISK

The first prerequisite for risk evaluation is the correct diagnosis of epilepsy. A good family history and pedigree are needed. In the family history, precise data are needed on the presence or absence of seizures in mother, father, siblings, and previous generations. A head trauma is often given by the patient as a cause of epilepsy. However, if the mother, father or sibling also has epilepsy, the possibility of a genetic aetiology should be considered. The sibling risk is higher when there is a parental positive seizure history both for epilepsy (7.4% versus 2.8%) and for seizures (12.3% versus 4.7%) (Anderson and Hauser, 1991). There seems to be a difference in the offspring risk for epilepsy between affected mother and fathers. The standardized morbidity ratio was 4.4 (95% CI 2.6–7.1) for offspring of affected mothers but only 1.6 (95% CI 0.6–3.6) for offspring of affected fathers (Ottman et al., 1988).

It is well known that most epilepsies have their onset before the age of 20 years. In the Comprehensive Epilepsy Program of Minnesota (Anderson and Hauser, 1991), the lower the age of the proband at onset of epilepsy, the higher the cumulative sibling risk by age 40 years. The differences might be greater if recall bias could be excluded. A large study (Ottman et al., 1995a) addressed the cumulative incidence from birth up to 40 years of age of epilepsy in parents, siblings and offspring and obtained the corresponding cumulative incidence rates of 1.8%, 2.9% and 5.6%. The differences, however, disappeared after controlling for age and birth year of the relatives, arguing for under-reporting in persons born in earlier time periods rather than for a real increase in incidence. The sibling risk for febrile convulsions and unprovoked seizures is higher than the average when the proband has febrile convulsions, unprovoked seizures or both (Table 6). The sibling risk for any seizures and for epilepsy is high, particularly when the proband's epilepsy had its onset before the age of 10 years (Table 7). The sibling risk is higher when the proband has an idiopathic epilepsy with generalized spike-and-wave discharges on the EEG compared with symptomatic epilepsy and focal EEG findings (Table 8).

Table 6. Sibling risk for febrile convulsions and unprovoked seizures.

Proband seizure	Total no. of siblings	Febrile convulsions (%)	Unprovoked seizures (%)
Febrile convulsions only	967	7.7	2.9
Unprovoked seizures only	552	4.5	2.9
Both febrile and unprovoked seizures	79	11.4	6.3

Source: Hauser *et al.*, 1985.

Table 7. Sibling risk for epilepsy by proband's age at onset of epilepsy.

Age at onset (years)	Seizures (%)	Epilepsy (%)
0–9	9.5	5.5
10–24	5.8	3.8
25–39	2.6	1.9

Source: Anderson and Hauser, 1990.

Table 8. Offspring risk for seizures and spike-and-wave EEG by type of proband epilepsy.

Type of proband epilepsy	Offspring epilepsy (%)	Offspring febrile convulsions (%)	Spike-and-wave (%)
Absence	6.7	10.0	63.6
Myoclonic petit mal	14.8	7.4	56.3
Awakening petit mal	4.8	11.1	44.8
Grand mal during sleep	2.0	2.0	28.0
Diffuse grand mal	6.3	1.6	33.3
Psychomotor	0.6	5.1	31.6
Focal	–	3.6	16.7

Source: Tsuboi, 1980.

Generalized tonic-clonic convulsions and simple and complex partial seizures, with or without secondary generalization, occur at all ages. In children and adolescents, the appearance of many other seizure types is dependent on age and, apparently, on developmental maturation of brain structures and biochemistry. Along with the cerebral maturation process, the phenotype of the seizures is also changing, for example from infantile spasms to Lennox–Gastaut syndrome and possibly further to secondary generalized partial seizures. Whatever the seizure type of the proband, the type of possible epileptic seizures or syndrome of siblings or offspring is more or less

Table 9. Sibling risk for any kind of seizure by type of EEG findings in relatives.

EEG finding in proband	No. of siblings	With any seizure (%)
Photosensitivity	43	7.0
Theta rhythms	24	12.5
Spike-and-wave during rest	20	35.0
Spike-and-wave plus photosensitivity and/or theta rhythms	27	33.3
Normal EEG	123	4.1

Source: Doose *et al.*, 1984.

unpredictable, though similarity to some extent can be found (Tsuboi, 1980). A risk for offspring epilepsy is 2–4% but is increased up to 5% when all risk factors are considered: onset at early age, occurrence of epilepsy in several relatives as generalized seizures and/or as generalized discharges on the EEG.

Certain abnormal EEG features are observed in relatives of the proband more often at certain ages than otherwise, suggesting a genetic determination of occurrence (Baier and Doose, 1987). These features include inter-ictal generalized spike-and-wave discharges and intermittent photostimulation, which each occur predominantly between 5 and 15 years, and a bilateral synchronous theta pattern, which is most often found in children aged 2–6 years (Table 9). Compared with normal EEG, the risk of any seizure was two- to threefold in the presence of photosensitivity in a sibling of an epilepsy proband with generalized minor seizures, and eight- to ninefold, when spike-and-wave pattern only or associated with photosensitivity and/or theta pattern (Doose *et al.*, 1984).

CONCLUSIONS

Mendelian inheritance works in the same way in the domain of epilepsy as in other diseases. However, this mode of inheritance is found in only 1–2% of epilepsies. So, the overwhelming majority of epilepsies are inherited in a non-Mendelian way, which means a virtually lower inheritability than in monogenic genetics. In the general population, the cumulative incidence of epilepsy is 1–2%. The sibling risk is only 2–3%, when the proband has epilepsy with partial seizures, but is 7–10% when the proband has childhood absence or other idiopathic generalized epilepsy. The sibling risk is still higher, 11–15%, when the proband or the sibling or both have generalized spike-and-wave EEG discharges. The overall risk to offspring is about 5%. It is higher if the mother is affected, when more than one family member is affected, and when the proband has early onset of seizures or generalized spike-and-wave discharges; it is lower if these risk factors are not present. In genetic counselling the sibling and family histories for epileptic seizures are of paramount importance. However, many variables remain in the counselling of individuals with epilepsy.

REFERENCES

Andermann, E. (1982). Multifactorial inheritance of generalized and focal epilepsy. In: Anderson, V.E., Hauser, W.A., Penry, J.K. *et al.* (Eds), *Genetic Basis of the Epilepsies*. Raven Press, New York, pp. 355–374.

Anderson, V.E. and Hauser, W.A. (1991). Genetics. In: Dam, M. and Gram, L. (Eds), *Comprehensive Epileptology*. Raven Press, New York, pp. 57–76.

Back, E., Voiculescu, I., Brunger, M. and Wolff, G. (1989). Familial ring (20) chromosome mosaicism. *Hum Genet* **83**, 148–154.

Baier, W.K. and Doose, H. (1987). Interdependence of different genetic EEG patterns in siblings of epileptic patients. *EEG Clin Neurophysiol* **66**, 483–488.

Bray, P. and Wiser, W.C. (1965). Hereditary characteristics of familial temporo-central focal epilepsy. *Pediatrics* **36**, 207–211.

Currier, R.D., Kooi, K.A. and Saidman, L.J. (1963). Prognosis of pure petit mal: a follow-up study. *Neurology* **13**, 959–967.

Delgado-Escueta, A.V., Greenberg, D., Weissbecker, K. *et al.* (1990). Gene mapping in the idiopathic generalized epilepsies. *Epilepsia* **31** (suppl 3), 519–529.

DiMauro, S., Ricci, E., Hirano, M., De Vivo, D.C. (1991). In: Anderson, V.E., Hauser, W.A., Leppik, I.E., Noebels, J.L. and Rich, S.S. (Eds), *Genetic Strategies in Epilepsy Research* (*Epil Res* (suppl 4).) Elsevier, Amsterdam, pp. 173–180.

Doose, H., Baier, W. and Reinsberg, E. (1984). Genetic heterogeneity of spike-wave epilepsies. In: Porter, R.J., Mattson, R.H., Ward, A.A. Jr and Dam, M. (Eds), *Advances in Epileptology: XVth Epilepsy International Symposium*. Raven Press, New York, pp. 515–519.

Gardiner, R.M. (1996). Genetics. In: Wallace, S. (Ed.), *Epilepsy in Children*. Chapman & Hall Medical, London, pp. 153–165.

Greenberg, D.A., Delgado-Escueta, A.V., Wideliz, H. *et al.* (1988). Juvenile myoclonic epilepsy may be linked to the BF and HLA loci human chromosome. *Am J Med Genet* **31**, 185–192.

Greenberg, D.A., Delgado-Escueta, A.V., Maldonade, H.M. *et al.* (1989). Segregation analysis of juvenile myoclonic epilepsy. In: Beck-Mannagetta, G., Anderson, V.E., Doose, H. and Janz, D. (Eds), *Genetics of the Epilepsies*. Springer-Verlag, Berlin, pp. 53–61.

Greenberg, D.A., Durner, M., Resor, S., Rosenbaum, D. and Shinnar, S. (1995). The genetics of idiopathic generalized epilepsies of adolescent onset: differences between juvenile myoclonic epilepsy and epilepsy with random grand mal and with awakening grand mal. *Neurology* **45**, 942–946.

Harbord, M.G., Hwang, P.A., Robinson, B.H., Becker, L.E., Hunjan, A. and Murphy, E.G. (1991). Infant-onset progressive myoclonus epilepsy. *J Child Neurol* **6**, 134–142.

Hauser, W.A. and Annegers, J.F. (1991). Risk factors for epilepsy. In: Anderson, V.E., Hauser, W.A., Leppik, I.E., Noebels, J.L. and Rich, S.S. (Eds), *Genetic Strategies in Epilepsy Research* (*Epil Res* (suppl 4).) Elsevier, Amsterdam, pp. 45–52.

Hauser, W.A., Annegers, J.F., Anderson, V.E. and Kurland, L.T. (1985). The risk of seizure disorders among relatives of children with febrile convulsions and unprovoked seizures. *Neurology* **35**, 1268–1273.

Hauser, W.A., Morris, M.L., Heston, L.L. *et al.* (1986). Seizures and myoclonus in patients with Alzheimer's disease. *Neurology* **36**, 1226–1230.

Heijbel, J., Blom, S., Rasmuson, M. *et al.* (1975). Benign epilepsy of childhood with centro-temporal EEG foci: a genetic study. *Epilepsia* **16**, 285–293.

Hirvasniemi, A., Lang, H., Lehesjoki, A.-E. and Leisti, J. (1994). Northern epilepsy syndrome. An inherited childhood onset epilepsy with associated mental deterioration. *J Med Genet* **31**, 177–182.

Holmes, G.L. (1987). Genetics in epilepsy. In: Holmes, G.L. (Ed.), *Diagnosis and Management of Seizures of Children*. Saunders, Philadelphia, PA, pp. 56–71.

Holopainen, I., Penttinen, M., Lakkala, T. and Äärimaa, T. (1994). Ring chromosome 20 mosaicism in a girl with complex partial seizures. *Dev Med Child Neurol* **36**, 70–73.

Lai, F. and Williams, R.S. (1989). A prospective study of Alzheimer disease in Down syndrome. *Arch Neurol* **46**, 849–853.

Lennox, W.G. (1951). Heredity of epilepsy as told by relatives and twins. *JAMA* **146**, 529–536.

Lugaresi, E., Pazzaglia, P., Guyot, M. *et al.* (1973). Evolution and prognosis of the petit mal absence type. In: Lugaresi, E., Pazzaglia, P. and Tassinara, C.A. (Eds), *Prognosis of Epilepsy*. Aulo Gaggi, Bologna, pp. 2–22.

McKusick, V.A. (1990). *Mendelian Inheritance in Man*. Johns Hopkins University Press, Baltimore, MD.

Metrakos, J.D. and Metrakos, K. (1972). *Genetic factors in the epilepsies*. In: *The Epidemiology of Epilepsy: A Workshop*. US Government Printing Office, Washington, DC, pp. 97–102.

Miettinen, O.S. (1985). *Theoretical Epidemiology. Principles of Occurrence Research in Medicine*. John Wiley, New York.

Montagna, P., Gallassi, R., Medori, R. *et al.* (1988). MELAS syndrome: characteristic migraineous and epileptic features and maternal transmission. *Neurology* **38**, 751–754.

Musumeci, S.A., Colognola, R.M. and Ferri, R. (1988). Fragile X syndrome: a particular epileptogenic EEG pattern. *Epilepsia* **29**, 41–47.

Norio, R. and Koskiniemi, M. (1979). Progressive myoclonus epilepsy: genetic and nosological aspects with special reference to 107 Finnish patients. *Clin Genet* **15**, 382–398.

Ottman, R., Annegers, J.F., Hauser, W.A. and Kurland, L.T. (1988). Higher risk of seizures in offspring of mothers than of fathers with epilepsy. *Am J Hum Genet* **43**, 257–264.

Ottman, R., Lee, J.H., Hauser, W.A. and Risch, N. (1995a). Birth cohort and familial risk of epilepsy: the effect of diminished recall in studies of lifetime prevalence. *Am J Epidemiol* **141**, 235–241.

Ottman, R., Risch, N., Hauser, W.A. *et al.* (1995b). Localization of a gene for partial epilepsy to chromosome 10q. *Nat Genet* **10**, 56–60.

Panayiotopoulos, C.P. and Obeid, T. (1989). Juvenile myoclonic epilepsy: an autosomal recessive disease. *Ann Neurol* **25**, 440–443.

Phillips, H.A., Scheffer, I.E., Bercovic, S.F., Hollway, G.E., Sutherland, G.R. and Mulley, J.C. (1995). Localization of a gene for autosomal dominant nocturnal frontal lobe epilepsy to chromosome 20q 13.2. *Nat Genet* **10**, 117–118.

Salonen, R., Somer, M., Haltia, M., Lorenz, M. and Norio, R. (1991). Progressive encephalopathy with edema, hypsarrhythmia, and optic atrophy (PEHO syndrome). *Clin Genet* **39**, 287–293.

Scheffer, I.E., Bhatia, K.P., Lopes-Cendes, I. *et al.* (1994). Autosomal dominant frontal epilepsy misdiagnosed as sleep disorder. *Lancet* **343**, 515–517.

Serratosa, J., Weisbecker, K. and Delgado-Escueta, A. (1990). Childhood absence epilepsy: an autosomal recessive disorder? *Epilepsia* **31**, 651.

Sillanpää, M., Koskenvuo, M., Romanov, K. and Kaprio, J. (1991). Genetic factors in epileptic seizures: evidence from a large twin population. *Acta Neurol Scand* **84**, 523–526.

Sim, M., Turner, E. and Smith, W.T. (1966). Cerebral biopsy in the investigation of presenile dementia. I. Clinical aspects. *Br J Psychiatry* **112**, 119–125.

Somer, M. (1993). The PEHO syndrome. Progressive encephalopathy with edema, hypsarrhythmia, and optic atrophy [Thesis]. Yliopistopaino, Helsinki.

Stafstrom, C.E. (1993). Epilepsy in Down syndrome: clinical aspects and possible mechanisms. *Am J Ment Retard* **98**, 12–26.

Tahvanainen, E., Ranta, S., Hirvasniemi, A. *et al.* (1994). The gene for a recessively inherited human childhood progressive epilepsy with mental retardation maps to the distal short arm of chromosome 8. *Proc Natl Acad Sci USA* **91**, 7267–7270.

Tsuboi, T. (1980). Genetic aspects of epilepsy. *Folia Psychiatr Neurol Jpn* **34**, 215–225.

Zonana, J., Silvey, K. and Strimling, B. (1984). Familial neonatal and infantile seizures: an autosomal-dominant disorder. *Am J Med Genet* **18**, 455–459.

Epilepsy and Pregnancy
Edited by T. Tomson, L. Gram, M. Sillanpää and S.I. Johannessen
© 1997 Wrightson Biomedical Publishing Ltd

20

Recommendations for the Management and Care of Pregnant Women with Epilepsy

TORBJÖRN TOMSON, LENNART GRAM,
MATTI SILLANPÄÄ AND SVEIN I. JOHANNESSEN

INTRODUCTION

Over recent years a group of clinician-investigators (Delgado-Escueta and Janz, 1992) and the Commission on Genetics, Pregnancy, and the Child of the International League Against Epilepsy (1989, 1993) have issued guidelines for the care of women of childbearing age with epilepsy. However, there is a need for updated recommendations because some new relevant knowledge has emerged and several new antiepileptic drugs have been introduced since then.

The present recommendations for the management of pregnant women with epilepsy include issues such as preconception and genetic counselling; treatment and care during pregnancy, delivery and puerperium; prenatal diagnosis; and the effect of maternal treatment on the newborn and breastfeeding. The guidelines reflect the authors' interpretations of the data presented in previous chapters of this volume to which the interested reader is referred for the original references.

PRECONCEPTION AND GENETIC COUNSELLING

Reproduction and sexual life may be affected in many different ways in the woman with epilepsy. Several forms of idiopathic epilepsy have a major genetic contribution. Hence, preconception and genetic counselling should be given to every epileptic woman of childbearing age. They should be counselled before conception and again during pregnancy. The following issues should be taken into account when counselling:

1) Problems with reproduction and sexual life may result from epilepsy, seizures, the underlying disorder, or treatment with antiepileptic drugs. Fertility tends to be reduced due to both social and medical reasons. The marriage rate and the number of own children are lower than in the general population. This is particularly the case in patients with associated handicaps. Antiepileptic medication may induce endocrine disorders affecting reproduction. Thus, to enhance fertility the use of antiepileptic drugs should be minimized. However, this ambition has to be balanced against the significant risk caused by generalized convulsions. Enzyme-inducing antiepileptic drugs may reduce the effect of oral contraceptive pills which may result in unexpected pregnancies.

2) Genetic counselling is complicated by the heterogeneity of epilepsy. Epilepsy may be an integral part of a Mendelian condition, such as inborn errors of metabolism and neurodegenerative disorders. In such cases it is often possible to make an accurate estimate of the offspring's risk of epilepsy. Genetic counselling is also relatively reliable in the case of idiopathic epilepsies for which the gene has been mapped, e.g. progressive myoclonus epilepsy or benign familial neonatal convulsions. When the primary cause of epilepsy is unknown, empiric recurrence risks have to be used taking into account the family history and the relationship between risks to sibs or offspring and age of onset of epilepsy in the proband. The empiric risk of having a child who will develop epilepsy, when one parent is affected, is about 5%. It is considerably higher if more than one family member has epilepsy.

3) Epilepsy is associated with an increased risk of major malformations. In addition, minor structural anomalies and a slightly elevated risk of impaired psychomotor development have been reported as results of intrauterine exposure to antiepileptic drugs, though data on this are scanty and partly conflicting. The overall chance of giving birth to a child without major malformations is 94–96%, compared with about 98% for the general population. The woman with epilepsy should be informed of these risks and of the option of prenatal diagnosis as discussed below.

4) Women of childbearing age with epilepsy should be informed about the general principles of antiepileptic drug use in pregnancy (see below). The importance of making any major change in drug therapy *before* pregnancy should be stressed. Women should be made aware that generalized convulsions during pregnancy can be hazardous to them and the fetus, and that seizures should therefore be well controlled from onset of pregnancy until delivery.

Information should also include recommendations concerning folate supplementation as outlined below:

• Any use of tobacco, alcohol and unnecessary drugs should be avoided.

- Close collaboration is needed between the family, the neurologist and the obstetrician, particularly when there are difficulties in balancing seizure control and pregnancy.

TREATMENT WITH ANTIEPILEPTIC DRUGS DURING PREGNANCY

A pregnant woman with epilepsy should be treated according to the usual therapeutic rules, i.e. whenever possible the woman should be controlled with a single antiepileptic drug, with the lowest effective dosage. With respect to the fetus it is, however, of particular importance to keep the pregnant woman free from tonic-clonic seizures. If possible all major changes in medication should be made before pregnancy. For valproate, two to three times daily dosing is recommended, preferably with a slow-release preparation, because the teratogenic effects are believed to result from high peak serum levels.

None of the drugs is known to cause less fetal abnormality than any other. If seizure control is satisfactory it is probably best to leave the treatment unchanged. None of the newer antiepileptic drugs (felbamate, gabapentin, lamotrigine, oxcarbazepine, topiramate and vigabatrin) is presently licensed for use in pregnancy.

At constant drug dosage the serum level of most antiepileptic drugs tends to decrease during pregnancy, but returns to prepregnancy level within the first month after delivery. This is of clinical importance because low serum levels may result in seizures. It is common practice to increase dosage according to the serum levels of antiepileptic drugs. However, given that the concentrations of individual drugs are affected differently by pregnancy and because the seizure frequency in pregnancy does not always correlate with antiepileptic drug serum levels, dosage adjustments have often been based on the clinical condition. Recent studies suggest that total carbamazepine serum levels are slightly lower during the third trimester as compared with baseline, whereas the unbound, pharmacologically active concentration remains essentially unchanged. In contrast, while total phenytoin serum levels decrease steadily as pregnancy progresses, unbound levels decrease far less. Total valproate serum levels also decrease as pregnancy proceeds, but the change in unbound concentrations may be insignificant. Serum levels of ethosuximide usually remain fairly constant during pregnancy.

Recent findings indicate that total serum levels may be misleading, and that monitoring of unbound concentrations may be advantageous during pregnancy. Thus, preferably both total and unbound serum levels should be closely monitored (once a month in patients with unstable seizure control, less frequently in well controlled patients) to determine the lowest effective dose and to avoid the harm of seizures and drugs to the mother and fetus. Monitoring unbound drug levels is, however, only relevant for highly protein-bound drugs such as phenytoin and valproate. Due to low unbound drug concentrations, sensitive and reliable analytical methods and quality control programmes are mandatory. After delivery, the serum levels should be monitored during the first month, since a dose reduction may be necessary to prevent toxicity.

A decrease in serum levels of antiepileptic drugs alone does not generally justify an increase in dose. The overall clinical state should be assessed. Ideally, the individual patient's optimal drug concentration and sensitivity to changes in drug levels should be known from before pregnancy and may thus be taken into account when changes in drug levels during pregnancy are evaluated. In addition to providing information of importance for therapeutic decisions, regular monitoring of antiepileptic drugs during pregnancy may enhance compliance with the prescribed drug therapy.

Summary of treatment strategy

- Use first-line drug for seizure type and epilepsy syndrome.
- Use monotherapy at lowest dose and serum level that protects against tonic-clonic seizures.
- If possible, avoid valproate and carbamazepine when there is a family history of neural tube defects.
- If possible, avoid polytherapy, especially a combination of valproate, carbamazepine and phenobarbital.
- Monitor serum levels of antiepileptic drugs regularly and, if available, unbound serum levels of phenytoin and valproate.
- In cases of valproate treatment, avoid high peak serum levels. Use a slow-release preparation given two to three times daily.

PRENATAL DIAGNOSIS

A malformation-directed ultrasound investigation should be offered to all patients at week 18–20. The sensitivity of the method depends on the experience of the investigator and should therefore be carried out by highly qualified sonographers. An expert sonographer will be able to detect more than 90% of neural tube defects (NTDs) at week 18–20. Skin-covered NTDs, not revealed by an increase in alfa-fetoprotein (AFP), can be reliably diagnosed or excluded. NTDs are generally associated with typical, recognizable changes in the fetal brain.

The majority of cleft lip and/or palates and heart anomalies can also be diagnosed by ultrasound at week 18–20 if performed by an expert.

Information on the occurrence of such malformations may be of value, although not leading to artificial abortion. In the future, a vaginal ultrasound at week 12–14 can be offered as an additional option.

Patients being treated with valproate and carbamazepine have an increased risk of giving birth to a child with an NTD (1–2% and 0.5–1.0%, respectively). They should therefore be counselled for amniocentesis at week 15–16 with determination of AFP in amniotic fluid. Counselling should include information on the advantages, limitations and risks of the method as compared with ultrasound. Amniocentesis has a somewhat higher sensitivity for detecting open NTDs, but will not detect those that are skin-covered. In addition, there is a 0.5–1.0% risk of abortion induced by amniocentesis.

Because of concern regarding the risk of abortion induced by amniocentesis, some mothers may prefer a combination of maternal serum AFP and malformation-directed ultrasonography. However, the sensitivity of AFP in maternal serum is only about 80% in NTD pregnancies.

The outlined recommendation for mothers treated with carbamazepine and valproate also applies to all new antiepileptic drugs since their teratogenic potential is largely unknown (see below).

Patients should be informed about the possibility of performing a chromosomal investigation on fetal cells if amniocentesis is carried out.

SUPPLEMENTATION WITH FOLATE AND OTHER VITAMINS

In general, the diet of all epileptic women of childbearing age should contain adequate amounts of folic acid. On the basis of existing studies of folate supplementation in healthy women and in women with epilepsy, before and during pregnancy, it is recommended that women with epilepsy have a daily intake of 0.4 mg of folate from the time they commence trying to become pregnant until the twelfth gestational week. The most practical way to achieve this is in the form of tablets of 0.4 mg given once daily.

If a woman has previously given birth to a child with a neural tube defect, the recommended daily folate supplement is 4 mg for the same time period as above. Some advocate a supplementation of 4 mg folate per day also for women treated with valproate or carbamazepine, since they have an equally increased risk of giving birth to a child with NTD. However, in this population documentation of an effect of high-dose folate supplementation on the risk of NTD in the offspring is lacking, and unknown adverse events of high-dose folate supplementation cannot be excluded.

All newborns should receive intramuscular injections of 1 mg of phytomenadione in order to avoid coagulation defects. In addition, a daily oral intake of 20 mg of vitamin K is sometimes recommended during the last month of pregnancy to women treated with enzyme-inducing antiepileptic drugs as well as regular oral vitamin K supplementation to the newborn for the first three months of life. However, there is no consensus concerning oral vitamin K supplementation.

LABOUR, DELIVERY AND THE OFFSPRING

Labour and delivery do not generally imply any particular obstetric measures, for example caesarean section. However, an increased risk of pregnancy-induced hypertension and preeclampsia, bleeding and preterm birth must be considered.

The risk for convulsions is 1–2% during labour and delivery. Serum concentrations of antiepileptic drugs should be determined at week 34–36 and the dose adjusted as necessary to cover the imminent delivery. Antiepileptic medication should be administered normally throughout labour and delivery to maintain adequate serum levels. In case of any doubts, serum concentrations should be determined daily and the dosage increased accordingly.

Administration of barbiturates or diazepam during the third trimester may cause newborn abstinence symptoms, such as irritability, hyperactivity, tremor, muscular hypertonia, tachypnoea, vomiting and poor weight gain.

Neonates born to mothers with clonazepam therapy may have severe sedation with apnoea, hypotonia and cyanosis for several hours after delivery. Administration of diazepam during delivery implies a risk of sedation of the newborn due to the rapid passage of the drug through the placenta and the slow metabolism of diazepam in the newborn.

BREAST-FEEDING

Any advice against nursing must be based on solid evidence since breast-feeding is the best way to feed a newborn infant and, furthermore, is of indisputable value for the development of a sound mother–child relationship.

Possible effects on the infant of antiepileptic drug exposure through breast-feeding depend on the amount of drug excreted in breast milk, and on the ability of the infant to eliminate the drug.

For phenytoin and valproate, drug exposure through breast milk is small. Serum concentrations of the drugs in the nursed infant are so low that no pharmacological effect can be expected, but dose-independent hypersensitivity reactions, though rare, cannot be excluded. There is no reason to discourage women treated with these drugs from breast-feeding, but the paediatrician should always consider the possibility of drug effects if abnormal signs or symptoms appear in the infant.

In breast-fed children of mothers on carbamazepine, phenobarbital, primidone, benzodiazepines or ethosuximide, drug concentrations may occasionally reach levels high enough to exert pharmacological effects. However, this does not warrant general advice against breast-feeding, but rather prompts a closer observation of the infant for drug effects. In the event of suspected side-effects, serum concentrations of the antiepileptic drugs should be determined in the infant.

There is a paucity of data on the excretion of new antiepileptic drugs in breast milk, and on the capacity of the infant to eliminate these drugs. Breast-feeding should therefore be monitored by analysis of the serum concentration in the infant, the drug concentration in the mother's breast milk and serum and by observation of possible drug effects in the infant.

NEW ANTIEPILEPTIC DRUGS AND PREGNANCY

All established major antiepileptic drugs (phenobarbital, phenytoin, carbamazepine, ethosuximide and valproate) have a teratogenic potential, irrespective of the mode of action of the drug, and despite a variable outcome of tests of reproduction toxicology. Some of the new drugs have a different profile in preclinical tests of reproduction toxicology, with no teratogenic effects in animals demonstrated for lamotrigine and gabapentin. However, the available clinical data on the use of these drugs in human pregnancy are very limited and mainly confined to new drugs used in combination with established antiepileptic drugs. The documentation is insufficient to allow conclusions on teratogenic potential and profile, and on the pharmacokinetics of the new drugs during pregnancy. Despite all precautions, an increasing number of women become pregnant while taking the new drugs. It is essential that the information from these pregnancies is compiled to form the basis for more rational future recommendations on the use of the new drugs during pregnancy. This needs to be done on a multicentre basis. Physicians responsible for treatment should therefore report all such cases to the international study which is initiated by the International League Against Epilepsy.

- A new antiepileptic drug should be used in pregnancy only if, in the opinion of the treating physician, the use of that specific drug is necessary to obtain seizure control.
- Patients treated with new antiepileptic drugs during pregnancy should be offered the same type of prenatal diagnosis as those patients treated with valproate or carbamazepine.
- Drug levels should preferably be monitored at monthly intervals throughout pregnancy, the main objective being to increase knowledge

of the kinetics of the new drugs in pregnancy rather than to guide dosage in the individual patient.

- The outcome of all pregnancies where new antiepileptic drugs have been used should be recorded according to a formal protocol and included in a prospective multicentre study, and also reported to the manufacturer.

REFERENCES

Commission on Genetics, Pregnancy, and the Child, International League Against Epilepsy (1989). Guidelines for the care of epileptic women of childbearing age. *Epilepsia* **30**, 409–410.

Commission on Genetics, Pregnancy, and the Child, International League Against Epilepsy (1993). Guidelines for the care of women of childbearing age with epilepsy. *Epilepsia* **34**, 588–589.

Delgado-Escueta, A.V. and Janz, D. (1992). Consensus guidelines: preconception counseling, management, and care of the pregnant woman with epilepsy. *Neurology* **42** (suppl 5), 149–160.

Index

209